SELF-ASSESSMENT IN
PHYSIOLOGY & PHARM

CW00846938

30, Albert
Grove.
Lenton.

SELF-ASSESSMENT IN
Physiology & Pharmacology

Terence Bennett
BSc, PhD, Reader

Sheila M. Gardiner
BSc, PhD, Lecturer

David R. Tomlinson
BSc, PhD, Senior Lecturer

All of the Department of Physiology and Pharmacology
The University of Nottingham Medical School

FOREWORD BY

W.C. Bowman and M.J. Rand

BLACKWELL SCIENTIFIC PUBLICATIONS

OXFORD LONDON EDINBURGH
BOSTON PALO ALTO MELBOURNE

© 1985 by
Blackwell Scientific Publications
Editorial offices:
Osney Mead, Oxford, OX2 0EL
8 John Street, London, WC1N 2ES
23 Ainslie Place, Edinburgh,
  EH3 6AJ
52 Beacon Street, Boston
  Massachusetts 02108, USA
744 Cowper Street, Palo Alto
  California 94301, USA
107 Barry Street, Carlton
  Victoria 3053, Australia

All rights reserved. No part of this
publication may be reproduced,
stored in a retrieval system, or
transmitted, in any form or by any
means, electronic, mechanical,
photocopying, recording or
otherwise without the prior
permission of the copyright owner

First published 1985

Set by Colset Pte. Ltd., Singapore
Printed and bound by
Billing & Sons Ltd, Worcester

DISTRIBUTORS

USA
  Blackwell Mosby Book
    Distributors
  11830 Westline Industrial Drive
  St Louis, Missouri 63141

Canada
  Blackwell Mosby Book
    Distributors
  120 Melford Drive, Scarborough
  Ontario M1B 2X4

Australia
  Blackwell Scientific Book
    Distributors
  31 Advantage Road, Highett
  Victoria 3190

British Library
Cataloguing in Publication Data

Bennett, Terence.
  Self-Assessment in Physiology
  and Pharmacology.
  1. Human physiology. —
  Problems, exercises, etc.
  2. Pharmacology. — Problems,
  exercises, etc.
  I. Title II. Gardiner, Sheila M.
  III. Tomlinson David R.
  612'.0076   QP40

ISBN 0–632–01161–0

Contents

*Subentries indicate the relating chapters and their contents in the
Textbook of Pharmacology.

Foreword

This book does not comprise the usual run-of-the-mill series of arbitrarily conceived multiple choice questions. Instead the questions are related to a particular textbook to which specific references are made, so that the student can easily find extra details that amplify the answers provided. This is surely a sound way to learn, as well as to assess one's progress. It is of course flattering for us that Drs Bennett, Gardiner and Tomlinson have chosen to key their questions to our textbook, but this aside the concept seems to be a worthy one. There is certainly no sycophantic acceptance that because it is in the book it must be correct. Where the textbook is out-of-date or in those instances (few we hope) where it is downright incorrect, Dr Bennett and his colleagues have given updated and amended answers, and we are grateful to them for this. It seems to us that their efforts may constitute the first of a new and welcome trend in self-assessment texts, and we congratulate them for thinking of it and wish them, and the students who use it, every success.

W.C. Bowman
Glasgow

M.J. Rand
Melbourne

Preface

This book is the result of the need for a self-assessment text concerning all the basic medical science aspects of physiology and pharmacology. In this way it differs from the books of multiple-choice questions on selected topics that are already available. More importantly, it places great emphasis on the background information to the questions in order that it should serve also as an effective teaching aid. To facilitate this function it is keyed into Bowman and Rand's *Textbook of Pharmacology* (Bowman W.C & Rand M.J. (1980) *Textbook of Pharmocology*, 2nd edition. Blackwell Scientific Publications, Oxford). Thus, together with the explanation of the answers to each question, chapter and page numbers are given in bold letters to indicate where more information may be obtained in the *Textbook of Pharmacology*. However, because the present text was not written in conjunction with the current edition of Bowman and Rand, there are some disparities between our statements and theirs. Where this occurs, the information in this book should be taken as correct.

We have arranged the material so that it corresponds to the systems courses of the basic medical sciences curriculum at The University of Nottingham Medical School in the order they are taught during the first six terms. However, it will be seen that this arrangement does not differ greatly from that of the *Textbook of Pharmacology*. We should be grateful to hear of any problems readers may encounter in using this book and of any suggestions that might prove helpful to future users.

Acknowledgements

We are grateful to our colleagues Geoff Bennett, Tony Birmingham, Jeff Fry, Ian Macdonald, Charles Marsden, John Patrick and Clive Wilson for their constructive criticisms of the typescript of this book, to Anne Brown (Blackwell Scientific Publications) for her help in the production of this book and to Peter Saugman (Blackwell Scientific Publications) without whose encouragement we would not have got this far. We are also indebted to Hazel Lee for the mammoth typing task she undertook, and to Rosemary Alefounder for being so tolerant when various difficult bits needed sorting out.

Cell Excitation

Q1 The membrane of the nerve axon:

   (a) comprises a lipid bilayer with protein on the inner and outer surfaces
   (b) contains an ATP-splitting enzyme which requires sodium and potassium ions for activity
   (c) actively extrudes sodium ions from the axoplasm
   (d) in the resting state, is more permeable to sodium than to potassium ions
   (e) is more permeable to lipophobic than to lipophilic substances

Q2 In the peripheral nervous system:

   (a) Schwann cells form the myelin sheaths around myelinated axons
   (b) the axons of unmyelinated fibres are not associated with Schwann cells
   (c) all autonomic efferent neurones have unmyelinated axons
   (d) the myelin lamellae forming the sheath are selectively impermeable to sodium ions
   (e) myelinated axons are free of myelin at the nodes of Ranvier

Q3 The velocity of conduction of a nerve action potential:

   (a) is inversely proportional to the cross-sectional area of the axon
   (b) is faster in a myelinated fibre than in a non-myelinated fibre of the same diameter
   (c) is decreased by cooling the nerve
   (d) may be 200 to 250 m/s in the fastest conducting mammalian fibres
   (e) is decreased by diseases which attack the myelin sheath

A1 (a) **T** The hydrophobic groups of the lipid bilayer are aligned in the centre of the membrane while the protein molecules are bound to the hydrophilic groups on the outer and inner surfaces   **2.4**

(b) **T** The result of activation is coupled sodium efflux and potassium influx — this is the sodium/potassium pump   **2.7, 5.5**

(c) **T** The sodium/potassium pump effectively extrudes sodium into the extracellular fluid, and maintains low intracellular levels of sodium   **2.7, 5.5**

(d) **F** The opposite is true; sodium ions are more hydrated than are potassium ions, thus there is a differential permeability (see (e))   **5.5**

(e) **F** The opposite is true; molecules of high lipid solubility dissolve in the membrane lipids and pass through   **2.5**

A2 (a) **T** The Schwann cell synthesizes and lays down the myelin around the axon   **5.2**

(b) **F** Unmyelinated fibres are invaginated into Schwann cells although the latter do not make myelin   **5.3**

(c) **F** Preganglionic fibres are myelinated, postganglionic fibres are usually unmyelinated   **9.4**

(d) **F** The myelin sheath is impermeable to all ions, thus saltatory conduction occurs by virtue of permeability changes where there is no myelin, i.e. at the nodes of Ranvier   **5.8**

(e) **T** Hence action potentials are generated only at the nodes (saltatory transmission)   **5.8**

A3 (a) **F** It is directly proportional to the cross-sectional area, because the greater the calibre of the axoplasm, the greater the internal current generated by the action potential. This increased current depolarizes the adjacent resting portions of membrane more rapidly, thus producing a greater conduction velocity   **5.3**

(b) **T** This is because action potentials are generated only at the nodes of Ranvier and transmission jumps the internodal regions (saltatory transmission)   **5.3**

(c) **T** The active stages of action potential generation are temperature sensitive since they are dependent on metabolic activity   **5.12**

(d) **F** Conduction velocity is never this high; 120 m/s is about the upper limit   **5.4**

(e) **T** Multiple sclerosis, for example, causes myelin loss which impairs saltatory transmission (see (b))   **5.2**

Q4 In the resting nerve axon:

    (a) a potential exists across the membrane such that the inside is negative with respect to the outside

    (b) the internal chloride ion concentration is higher than that outside

    (c) the axoplasm contains more negative charge in the form of organic anion than does the extracellular fluid

    (d) the transmembrane potential is close to the potassium equilibrium potential

    (e) elevation of the external potassium ion concentration would increase the magnitude of the transmembrane potential

Q5 The nerve action potential:

    (a) commences with a brisk increase in the permeability of the plasma membrane to sodium ions

    (b) comprises a depolarization, then a transient reversal of transmembrane potential, followed by repolarization

    (c) has a repolarization phase which is achieved by efflux of sodium ions

    (d) is followed by a period during which the nerve fibre is hyperexcitable

    (e) is generated only at the nodes of Ranvier in myelinated fibres

Q6 An excitatory postsynaptic potential (EPSP):

    (a) is itself propagated by the postsynaptic cell

    (b) comprises depolarization of the membrane to zero, transient reversal of potential, and then repolarization

    (c) is related in amplitude to the concentration of the initiating transmitter at the postsynaptic membrane

    (d) may summate both temporally and spatially with other EPSPs

    (e) is reduced in amplitude by drugs which block the postsynaptic receptors for the transmitter substance

A4 (a) **T** This resting membrane potential can be recorded with a microelectrode; it is usually 60 to 80 mV   **5.5**

(b) **F** The opposite is true; chloride ions are disposed such that their concentration gradient is balanced by the electrical gradient across the membrane   **5.5**

(c) **T** Many intracellular macromolecules carry dissociated carboxyl groups (i.e. cationic charges)   **5.5, 2.10**

(d) **T** The potassium equilibrium potential may be calculated fom the Nernst equation (see p. **2.11**) and compared with the measured resting potential   **5.5**

(e) **F** The opposite is true; when external potassium concentration rises the potassium equilibrium potential is shifted by entry of potassium ions, thus the inside becomes less negative with respect to the outside   **5.5**

A5 (a) **T** This is probably activated by calcium ions opening conductance channels for sodium ions   **5.7**

(b) **T** This describes the phenomenon recorded by a microelectrode   **5.7**

(c) **F** Efflux of potassium ions (due to increased potassium permeability) causes repolarization   **5.7**

(d) **F** The refractory period is due to reduced sodium permeability and increased potassium permeability leading to hypoexcitability   **5.9**

(e) **T** It is only at the nodes that the absence of myelin permits ion fluxes to occur   **5.8**

A6 (a) **F** An isolated EPSP is subthreshold and is not propagated   **5.20**

(b) **F** This describes the action potential. The EPSP is a depolarization of less than 10 mV   **5.20**

(c) **T** Amplitude increases with increasing transmitter concentration   **5.20**

(d) **T** Temporal summation (due to repeated activation of the same presynaptic element) and spatial summation (due to concurrent activation of different presynaptic elements) may cause suprathreshold depolarization and action potential initiation   **5.20**

(e) **T** The EPSP is generated as a consequence of interaction between the transmitter and its postsynaptic receptors, thus antagonism of this process reduces EPSP amplitude or even prevents the generation of the EPSP   **5.20**

Q7 The release of an excitatory synaptic transmitter from a nerve ending:

(a) is stimulated by the arrival of an action potential at the nerve terminal

(b) does not occur in the absence of extracellular calcium ions

(c) causes an increase in the permeability of the post-junctional membrane to chloride ions

(d) following electrical stimulation, occurs by exocytosis from synaptic vesicles

(e) may be followed by the transmitter acting on the pre-synaptic membrane to modulate further release

Q8 Local anaesthetic drugs:

(a) are selective towards large, rather than small diameter fibres

(b) are selective towards sensory, rather than motor fibres

(c) act on the nerve cell membrane to prevent the opening of some of the ion channels involved in the action potential

(d) may be given in combination with a vasoconstrictor to restrict and prolong their effect

(e) enhance myocardial excitability

Q9 Lignocaine:

(a) is hydrolysed by plasma esterases and so has a very brief action

(b) is approximately half as potent as procaine

(c) suppresses ventricular arrhythmias

(d) does not cross the blood–brain barrier

(e) may be given by epidural infusion to produce epidural anaesthesia

A7 (a) **T** This is the normal physiological process; nerve terminal depolarization increases calcium permeability, the influx of which triggers the exocytosis 5.22

(b) **T** Although some drugs (e.g. indirectly acting sympatho-mimetics) can evoke release without calcium, the arrival of a presynaptic action potential requires calcium for transmitter release 5.21

(c) **F** This would cause postsynaptic inhibition since chloride ions would move down their concentration gradient into the cell and hence hyperpolarize the postjunctional membrane 5.21

(d) **T** There is ultrastructural evidence that vesicles coalesce with the presynaptic membrane forming a pore through which the vesicle contents can enter the cleft 10.5, 10.6

(e) **T** This is well established for noradrenergic transmission where there is α_2-adrenoceptor-mediated inhibitory feedback on release and β-adrenoceptor-mediated facilitation 11.21

A8 (a) **F** Small diameter fibres are more readily affected, thus fibres which relay pain sensation (generally small dia-meter) tend to be affected when motor nerves (generally larger diameter) are not 16.30

(b) **F** The effect described above is not due to selectivity of action, thus sensory and motor axons of the same dia-meter are equally susceptible 16.30

(c) **T** Their action can be antagonized by increasing external sodium concentration. They also reduce the rise in potas-sium permeability that normally occurs during the action potential 5.16

(d) **T** The vasoconstrictor reduces local perfusion and so impairs absorption into the systemic circulation 16.36

(e) **F** They tend to reduce it; drugs such as lignocaine, which has many quinidine-like effects, are used as anti-arrhythmics 22.58

A9 (a) **F** Procaine is hydrolysed by plasma esterases, lignocaine is not, and was therefore introduced as a drug with a longer duration of action 16.35

(b) **F** Lignocaine is about twice as potent as procaine, possibly as a consequence of its resistance to hydrolysis in plasma (see above) 16.35

(c) **T** This occurs by stabilization of the membranes of ventri-cular ectopic pacemaker cells 22.58

(d) **F** Lignocaine, given systemically, enters the brain and depresses central nervous functions. It has been used to suppress convulsions 16.36

(e) **T** Lignocaine is one of several agents which may be so used 16.31

Introduction to the Nervous System

Q10 In the autonomic nervous system of man:

(a) sympathetic preganglionic cell bodies lie in the intermediolateral columns of the spinal cord between segments C1 to L3

(b) there are no discrete parasympathetic ganglia

(c) more than 80% of the postganglionic neurones are unmyelinated

(d) all preganglionic sympathetic neurones synapse in paravertebral ganglia

(e) preganglionic parasympathetic neurones in the Edinger-Westphal nucleus innervate cell bodies in the ciliary ganglion

Q11 In man, activation of the:

(a) sympathetic innervation of the stomach causes inhibition of gastric secretion

(b) parasympathetic innervation of the pancreas stimulates insulin release

(c) sympathetic innervation of the spleen causes contraction of the capsular smooth muscle

(d) parasympathetic innervation of the bladder causes relaxation of the detrusor muscle

(e) sympathetic innervation of the kidney causes release of renin

A10 (a) **F** Sympathetic preganglionic cell bodies are not found in   **9.1**
the cervical segments, only in segments T1 to L3

 (b) **F** Many postganglionic parasympathetic neurones form   **9.4**
ganglia in the cranial region

 (c) **T** Where they run together, as in the grey rami communi-   **9.2**
cantes, the absence of myelin is macroscopically
apparent (hence the grey colouration)

 (d) **F** Many synapse in prevertebral (i.e. coeliac, mesenteric   **9.2**
or hypogastric) plexuses, and some synapse with
adrenal medullary chromaffin cells

 (e) **T** These postganglionic cells innervate the constrictor   **9.3**
pupillae and the ciliary muscle; the axons are myeli-
nated (Group B)

A11 (a) **F** There is no evidence for a sympathetic inhibitory inner-   **9.7**
vation of the gastric mucosa. Sympathetic stimulation
causes inhibition of motility, sphincter contraction and
vasoconstriction

 (b) **T** The parasympathetic innervation of the islet β cells is   **9.7,**
excitatory and blocked by atropine (there are also α-   **19.50**
adrenoceptors that inhibit and β-adrenoceptors that
stimulate insulin release). It is probable that neural
mechanisms are involved in the fine control of insulin
release

 (c) **T** This effect is mediated via α-adrenoceptors. The splenic   **9.7,**
sinusoids act as a reservoir from which blood may be   **23.3**
shifted when needed (haemorrhage, exercise) but this
effect is less marked in man than in the dog, for example

 (d) **F** Parasympathetic stimulation causes contraction of the   **9.7,**
detrusor muscle and the longitudinal muscle around the   **27.20**
bladder neck and urethral orifice. This forces urine into
the urethra (the effect is enhanced by increased
abdominal pressure); inhibition of the external sphincter
permits voiding

 (e) **T** There is a direct innervation of the granular cells of the   **9.7**
juxtaglomerular apparatus; noradrenaline release acti-
vates β-adrenoceptors and stimulates renin release.
Sympathetic stimulation may also augment renin release
by causing a reduction in renal perfusion pressure

Q12 In man, activation of the:

(a) sympathetic innervation of the iris causes pupillodilatation

(b) parasympathetic innervation of salivary glands causes a sparse, mucinous secretion

(c) parasympathetic innervation of the lung causes bronchoconstriction only

(d) sympathetic innervation of the heart may cause shortening of the P–Q interval

(e) sympathetic innervation of the liver causes glycogenesis

Q13 In man, activation of the sympathetic innervation of:

(a) the adrenal medulla causes release of adrenaline and noradrenaline

(b) the genitalia causes erection

(c) eccrine sweat glands causes sweating which is inhibited by atropine

(d) skeletal muscle blood vessels may cause vasodilatation

(e) skeletal muscle blood vessels may cause vasoconstriction

A12 (a) **T** The sympathetic innervation of the radial muscles of the   **9.7,**
iris causes contraction (mediated via α-adrenoceptors)   **9.17**
of the fibres, thus increasing the diameter of the pupil

(b) **F** Stimulation of the parasympathetic innervation causes a   **9.7**
profuse watery secretion high in α-amylase (due to activation of the serous cells). Secretion is accompanied by
vasodilatation in the gland that is resistant to atropine; it
is possible the vasodilatation is due to release of vaso-
active intestinal polypeptide

(c) **F** As well as causing bronchoconstriction, activation of   **9.7**
parasympathetic fibres to the lung increases bronchial
mucosal secretion. Pre-medication with atropine serves
to suppress bronchial secretions during surgery (muscarinic effect)

(d) **T** Sympathetic fibres innervate myocardial and nodal and   **9.7**
conducting tissues. Conduction through the atrioventri-
cular node is relatively slow and thus it is responsible for
a large part of the P–Q interval. Sympathetic stimulation
increases conduction velocity and shortens the P–Q
interval (β_1 effect largely)

(e) **F** Noradrenaline (acting on β_2-adrenoceptors) stimulates   **9.7**
hepatic glycogenolysis and gluconeogenesis (from lac-
tate) and hence increases blood glucose

A13 (a) **T** The chromaffin cells receive a preganglionic innervation   **9.7**
from fibres in the splanchnic nerves. The acetylcholine
released acts on nicotinic receptors on the chromaffin
cells; the majority (about 80%) of these cells synthesize
and release adrenaline

(b) **F** Erection results from parasympathetically induced   **9.7,**
penile vasodilatation which leads to the erectile tissue   **20.24**
becoming filled with blood. Sympathetic stimulation
causes contraction of the epididymides, vasa deferentia,
seminal vesicles and prostate glands and detumescence
due to vasoconstriction in the penis

(c) **T** Eccrine sweat glands receive a sympathetic cholinergic   **9.7**
innervation which stimulates (via muscarinic receptors)
the glandular and myoepithelial cells

(d) **T** In man there is evidence for a sympathetic vasodilator   **9.7,**
innervation of precapillary arterioles. Acetylcholine   **23.14**
released acts on muscarinic receptors; this mechanism
is activated during the vasovagal response and, possibly,
at the onset of exercise

(e) **T** Skeletal muscle blood vessels also receive a noradrener-   **9.7,**
gic innervation. Noradrenaline acting on postjunctional   **23.14**
α_1- (and, possibly, α_2-)adrenoceptors causes vasoconstriction

Q14 In cholinergic autonomic neurones:

(a) synthesis of acetylcholine is dependent on the enzyme choline hydroxylase
(b) choline is synthesized in the cell body
(c) there is a high affinity transport mechanism which shifts choline from extracellular fluid into axoplasm
(d) hemicholiniums inhibit the synthesis of acetylcholine
(e) triethylcholine inhibits the synthesis of acetylcholine

Q15 In cholinergic autonomic neurones:

(a) acetylcholine is synthesized in the cell body and is transported to the nerve terminals in vesicles
(b) action potentials induce release of acetylcholine by a calcium-dependent process
(c) acetylcholine release may be facilitated by botulinum toxins
(d) acetylcholine release may be decreased by morphine
(e) acetylcholine release may be facilitated by noradrenaline

Q16 The action of acetylcholine:

(a) on the iris is mimicked by pilocarpine
(b) on the heart is antagonized by methacholine
(c) on the gut is mimicked by carbamylcholine (carbachol)
(d) on the bladder is antagonized by bethanechol
(e) on cutaneous blood vessels is antagonized by furtrethonium

A14 (a) **F** Acetylcholine is synthesized from choline and acetyl-coenzyme A — a reaction catalysed by choline acetyltransferase   10.1

(b) **F** Choline incorporated into acetylcholine is derived from extracellular fluid; some is derived from the diet but most is synthesized by the liver   10.1

(c) **T** This is distinct from the low affinity transport mechanism for choline possessed by most cells (to supply substrate for phospholipid synthesis)   10.1

(d) **T** They do so by competing with choline for the high affinity transport mechanism, and hence reducing choline availability for incorporation into acetylcholine   10.3

(e) **T** Triethylcholine, like hemicholinium 3, blocks choline transport and, in high doses, blocks postsynaptic acetylcholine receptors in autonomic ganglia   10.4

A15 (a) **F** Vesicles are probably synthesized in the cell body and transported to the terminals, but the acetylcholine contained in them is largely synthesized after the vesicles have reached the terminals   10.5

(b) **T** The action potential increases Ca^{2+} permeability and Ca^{2+} enters the axoplasm; it is possible that exocytosis involves Ca^{2+} activation of actin- and myosin-like proteins in the axoplasm   10.5

(c) **F** These toxins block the release of acetylcholine without affecting nerve conduction, acetylcholine synthesis, cholinesterase or cholinergic receptors; the effect is probably due to combination with the membrane lipids   10.7

(d) **T** An effect clearly demonstrated in postganglionic cholinergic terminals in the myenteric plexus, and providing evidence for the existence of prejunctional opiate receptors   10.8

(e) **F** Noradrenaline and other α-adrenoceptor agonists inhibit acetylcholine release by a prejunctional mechanism   10.8

A16 (a) **T** Topical pilocarpine causes miosis, and is used in the treatment of glaucoma   10.9

(b) **F** Methacholine mimics the action of acetylcholine on the heart, and may be used to terminate supraventricular tachycardias   10.10

(c) **T** Carbachol may be used to produce motility of the gut in postoperative adynamic ileus   10.10

(d) **F** Bethanechol, another parasympathomimetic, may be used to cause bladder contraction in non-obstructive urinary retention   10.10

(e) **F** Furtrethonium would cause a vasodilatation as does acetylcholine, although the former is used primarily to treat urinary retention in non-obstructive disorders   10.10

Introduction to the Nervous System   15

Q17 The pharmacological effects of atropine in man may include:

(a) an initial bradycardia when the administered dose is low

(b) cutaneous vasodilatation when given in large doses

(c) suppression of gastric acid secretion in response to a meal

(d) a reduction in intraocular pressure

(e) reduction in gastrointestinal motility

Q18 Atropine and/or hyoscine may be used clinically as:

(a) preoperative medications to inhibit bronchial secretions

(b) a means of reducing intraocular pressure

(c) bronchodilators

(d) prophylactic treatment for motion sickness

(e) routine treatment for peptic ulcer

A17 (a) **T**   Although attributed to a central stimulant action on   **10.12**
        medullary vagal centres, this effect is more likely due to
        an initial agonistic activity on cardiac muscarinic
        receptors

   (b) **T**   An effect unconnected with antimuscarinic activity and   **10.12**
        possibly due to a direct vasodilator action or to histamine
        release; 'atropine blush' is seen in atropine toxicity

   (c) **F**   Gastric acid secretion is stimulated by the vagi, although   **10.12**
        other factors (e.g. gastrin, histamine) predominate in the
        control of gastric acid secretion. Hence, when secretion
        is effected by the presence of food in the stomach
        atropine would not cause blockade

   (d) **F**   Atropine dilates the pupil (and paralyses the ciliary   **10.12**
        muscle); in older people, contraction of the iris into the
        angle of the anterior chamber blocks drainage and acute
        glaucoma may result

   (e) **T**   The vagal and sacral parasympathetic efferent outputs   **10.12**
        to the gut are antagonized by atropine, resulting in rela-
        tive gastrointestinal stasis

A18 (a) **T**   Bronchial secretion is stimulated by vagal activity acting   **10.13**
        through muscarinic receptors; excessive secretion might
        impair respiration; the sedative action of hyoscine is also
        useful preoperatively

   (b) **F**   Both drugs cause pupillodilatation and may cause an   **10.14**
        increase in intraocular pressure; the mydriasis they
        cause facilitates retinal examination

   (c) **T**   In some asthmatic patients antimuscarinic drugs may   **10.14**
        cause bronchodilatation (by antagonizing vagal efferent
        effects), although the muscarinic blocker, ipratropium,
        which may be given by inhalation would be preferred

   (d) **T**   Hyoscine has a good prophylactic effect against motion   **10.14**
        sickness — presumably attributable to its central
        depressant actions

   (e) **F**   The doses required to have any effect on gastric acid   **10.14**
        secretion are so great that side-effects predominate;
        furthermore, the reduction in gastric secretion volume
        may cause a rise in gastric acidity

Q19 Transmission through autonomic ganglia is impaired by:

(a) atropine
(b) hemicholinium
(c) hexamethonium
(d) decamethonium
(e) mecamylamine

Q20 Anticholinesterase drugs may be used:

(a) in the treatment of glaucoma
(b) to antagonize the effects of the neuromuscular blocking drug suxamethonium
(c) to antagonize the effects of the neuromuscular blocking drug, tubocurarine
(d) as therapy in myasthenia gravis
(e) as antihypertensive agents

Q21 The biosynthesis of noradrenaline:

(a) is dependent on the dietary intake of phenylalanine
(b) is inhibited by a variety of tyrosine analogues
(c) involves generation of large amounts of dihydroxyphenylalanine (dopa) intraneuronally
(d) involves the production of dopamine within the transmitter storage vesicles
(e) is inhibited by drugs that inhibit the vesicular uptake mechanism

A19	(a)	F	Although there are muscarinic receptors on postganglionic cell bodies, normal transmission appears to involve only nicotinic receptors	10.20
	(b)	T	Hemicholinium impairs preganglionic release of acetylcholine and hence interferes with transmission	10.21
	(c)	T	Hexamethonium is a non-depolarizing antagonist of postganglionic nicotinic receptors and thus interferes with ganglionic nicotinic transmission	10.22
	(d)	F*	Although a bisquaternary ammonium compound like hexamethonium, decamethonium is a depolarizing neuromuscular antagonist with little effect on ganglionic nicotinic receptors	10.22
	(e)	T	Mecamylamine blocks ganglionic nicotinic receptors in a non-competitive manner — possibly partly due to an intracellular action depressing sensitivity to acetylcholine	10.24

A20	(a)	T	Such drugs cause pupilloconstriction (by facilitating cholinergic transmission) and hence reduce intraocular pressure	10.35
	(b)	F	Suxamethonium is rapidly hydrolysed by cholinesterase; anticholinesterase would inhibit this effect and hence prolong the blockade	17.46
	(c)	T	Tubocurarine is a competitive antagonist for nicotinic receptors; anticholinesterases would increase the number of acetylcholine molecules available to compete with it	10.35
	(d)	T	Drugs such as pyridostigmine are useful in ameliorating the neuromuscular failure (due to nicotinic receptor antibodies) seen in myasthenia gravis	10.35
	(e)	F	At high doses, such drugs may exert acetylcholine-like effects, but vasodilatation is not commonly seen with usual doses	10.36

A21	(a)	F	Generally the dietary intake of tyrosine (derived from protein) suffices for noradrenaline synthesis	11.1
	(b)	T	These substances compete with tyrosine at the active centre of tyrosine hydroxylase — the rate-limiting step in noradrenaline synthesis	11.2
	(c)	F	Normally dopa does not accumulate in noradrenergic nerves since it is formed only slowly, and is rapidly converted to dopamine by dopa decarboxylase	11.2
	(d)	F	The production of dopamine depends on the action of dopa decarboxylase — an enzyme that is not associated with any subcellular structure; the dopamine formed in the cytoplasm is taken up into the storage vesicles	11.2
	(e)	T	Axoplasmic dopamine is taken up by the vesicular mechanism and is converted to noradrenaline by the enzyme dopamine-β-hydroxylase, found in the vesicles	11.3

Introduction to the Nervous System 19

Q22 In noradrenergic autonomic neurones:

(a) tyrosine hydroxylase is the rate-limiting enzyme in the synthetic pathway for noradrenaline

(b) the conversion of dopa to dopamine is inhibited competitively by carbidopa

(c) dopamine-β-hydroxylase is associated with mitochondria

(d) α-methyl dopa may be converted to α-methylnoradrenaline

(e) phenylethanolamine-N-methyltransferase is synthesized in the cell bodies and transported to the nerve terminals

Q23 In man, the degradation of catecholamines:

(a) may produce 3-methoxy compounds, which are biologically inactive

(b) may occur intraneuronally

(c) may occur in the gut

(d) may be impaired by pargyline

(e) is the most important mechanism in curtailing their biological action

Q24 Monoamine oxidase inhibitors:

(a) interfere specifically with the catabolism of noradrenaline

(b) lead to increases in the monoamine content of some brain and peripheral tissues

(c) may cause impairment of peripheral noradrenergic transmission

(d) may inhibit the actions of indirectly acting sympathomimetic amines

(e) potentiate the actions of exogenous noradrenaline

A22 (a) **T**   The rate of synthesis of tyrosine hydroxylase is increased when release rate is high (presumably due to reduction in end-product feedback inhibition) and vice versa   **11.2**

     (b) **T**   Carbidopa is used clinically to prevent peripheral decarboxylation of dopa administered in Parkinsonism, thereby permitting a lower dose of dopa to be employed   **11.2**

     (c) **F**   Dopamine-β-hydroxylase is associated with the storage vesicles; the conversion of dopamine to noradrenaline occurs within these   **11.3**

     (d) **T**   This is thought to be the mode of action of this antihypertensive drug — the α-methylnoradrenaline acting as a false transmitter   **11.3**

     (e) **F**   PNMT occurs in adrenaline-synthesizing chromaffin cells and neurones but is absent from noradrenergic neurones   **11.3**

A23 (a) **F**   Catechol-O-methyltransferase, acting on noradrenaline and adrenaline, produces normetanephrine and metanephrine which are inhibitors of catecholamine uptake into effector tissues (uptake 2)   **11.5**

     (b) **T**   Monoamine oxidase activity is associated with mitochondria in the axoplasm; catecholamines not within storage vesicles may be acted upon by this enzyme   **11.6**

     (c) **T**   Monoamine oxidase levels are particularly high in the intestinal mucosa and liver where the enzyme is involved in the degradation of dietary amines and those formed by bacterial action in the gut   **11.6**

     (d) **T**   Pargyline is a monoamine oxidase inhibitor that causes increased intraneuronal monoamine levels   **11.10**

     (e) **F**   About 80% of released noradrenaline is taken back into noradrenergic nerves in its original form   **11.14**

A24 (a) **F**   MAO inhibitors also interfere with liver microsomal enzymes, and hence are liable to potentiate the effects of drugs normally metabolized by this system (e.g. barbiturates, morphine, phenothiazines, tricyclic antidepressants)   **11.9**

     (b) **T**   It is possible that the increase in brain amines leads to their enhanced availability as transmitters and hence amelioration of depression   **11.9**

     (c) **T**   Treatment with MAO inhibitors leads to increased levels of tyramine and octopamine in noradrenergic nerves; these may act as false transmitters and thus impair transmission   **11.9**

     (d) **F**   Inhibition of MAO in the gut permits dietary amines to gain access to the circulation thereby enhancing their action; inhibition of liver microsomal enzymes potentiates the actions of other sympathomimetic amines   **11.10**

     (e) **F**   Neuronal uptake, rather than catabolism by MAO, is primarily responsible for terminating the action of noradrenaline   **11.10**

Q25 The uptake of noradrenaline:

  (a) into noradrenergic nerves is inhibited by reserpine
  (b) into noradrenergic nerves is inhibited by cocaine
  (c) by non-neuronal cells is inhibited by steroids
  (d) into noradrenergic nerves is inhibited by tricyclic antidepressant drugs
  (e) into noradrenergic nerves is inhibited by normetanephrine

Q26 The uptake of noradrenaline:

  (a) by storage vesicles is inhibited by reserpine
  (b) by noradrenergic nerves is dependent on a supply of ATP
  (c) by noradrenergic nerves is reduced by indirectly acting sympathomimetic amines
  (d) by non-neuronal tissue is inhibited by phenoxybenzamine
  (e) by noradrenergic neurones is inhibited by noradrenergic-neurone-blocking drugs

Q27 The release of noradrenaline from noradrenergic nerves:

  (a) is markedly increased by reserpine
  (b) may be reduced by acetylcholine
  (c) may be reduced by noradrenaline
  (d) is a calcium independent process
  (e) by reflex activation is accompanied by release of dopamine-β-hydroxylase

A25 (a) **F** Reserpine inhibits the vesicular uptake process not the axonal uptake process; it does so by competing with noradrenaline   **11.13**

(b) **T** The inhibition of neuronal uptake is independent of its local anaesthetic action and is responsible for the enhancement of responses to nerve stimulation accompanied by abolition of effects of indirect sympathomimetics   **11.17**

(c) **T** Cortisol has this effect *in vitro* and *in vivo* and thus enhances the action of indirect sympathomimetics   **11.20**

(d) **T** Desipramine is a particularly potent inhibitor of neuronal uptake; it is not known for certain if this is the basis of the action of tricyclic antidepressants in the central nervous system   **11.18**

(e) **F** Normetanephrine (formed from noradrenaline through the action of catechol-O-methyltransferase) is a potent inhibitor of extraneuronal uptake, but not of neuronal uptake   **11.20**

A26 (a) **T** The affinity of reserpine for the vesicular uptake mechanism is about 10 000 times greater than that of noradrenaline; high doses of reserpine irreversibly damage the storage vesicles   **11.13**

(b) **T** The uptake (uptake$_1$) is inhibited if both aerobic and anaerobic energy-yielding processes are inhibited   **11.15**

(c) **T** Substances such as tyramine inhibit neuronal uptake by competing for the transport mechanism but also displace noradrenaline from within the nerves   **11.17**

(d) **T** In addition to blocking neuronal uptake and α-adrenoceptors, phenoxybenzamine is a potent inhibitor of extraneuronal uptake   **11.19**

(e) **T** Guanethidine and related drugs compete for the axonal uptake mechanism, and hence also inhibit the effect of indirectly acting sympathomimetic amines   **11.18**

A27 (a) **F** Reserpine prevents vesicular binding of noradrenaline so the axoplasmic noradrenaline is attacked by monoamine oxidase; thus, following reserpine, metabolites are released   **11.14**

(b) **T** Prejunctional muscarinic receptors inhibit noradrenaline release; this effect may be important physiologically   **11.21**

(c) **T** Prejunctional α_2-adrenoceptors inhibit noradrenaline release; thus released noradrenaline has a negative feedback effect on further release   **11.21**

(d) **F** Exocytosis is a calcium-dependent process possibly involving calcium activation of axoplasmic contractile proteins   **11.20**

(e) **T** Dopamine-β-hydroxylase is present in the storage vesicles; its release along with noradrenaline and ATP supports the notion of exocytosis   **11.20**

Q28 Noradrenergic neurone blocking drugs such as guanethidine:

(a) are antagonized by drugs that inhibit neuronal uptake of amines

(b) act by depleting noradrenaline from intraneuronal stores

(c) have local anaesthetic activity

(d) may cause failure of ejaculation

(e) have a ganglion-blocking effect in isolated preparations

Q29 In a conscious human subject, intravenous injection of:

(a) noradrenaline would cause a rise in diastolic blood pressure

(b) noradrenaline may cause a bradycardia

(c) adrenaline, in moderate doses, would cause a rise in diastolic blood pressure

(d) adrenaline, in moderate doses, would cause a bradycardia

(e) dopamine would cause increased renal blood flow

A28 (a) **T**   Drugs such as cocaine, dexamphetamine and tricyclic   **11.24**
antidepressants antagonize the onset of action and
reverse the blockade once established

    (b) **F**   Doses just sufficient to cause transmission failure do not   **11.24**
cause depletion; any depletion seen is not due to libera-
tion of noradrenaline from vesicles but probably to a
transient reflex activation of neuronal activity

    (c) **T**   It has been suggested that high intraneuronal levels   **11.25**
block transmission due to a local anaesthetic action, pos-
sibly exerted at points of axonal branching

    (d) **T**   Due to inhibition of transmission from the sympathetic   **23.44**
nerves supplying the epididymis, vas deferens, seminal
vesicles and prostate gland

    (e) **T**   This effect *in vitro* is as powerful as that of many gan-   **11.25**
glion-blocking drugs; they also impair neuromuscular
transmission

A29 (a) **T**   Noradrenaline causes an increase in total peripheral   **11.28**
resistance due to α-adrenoceptor-mediated vasocon-
striction

    (b) **T**   Noradrenaline has a direct positive chronotropic action   **11.28**
but normally the rise in systemic arterial blood pressure
which it elicits causes a vagally mediated reflex
bradycardia

    (c) **F**   Except in large doses, adrenaline causes dilatation of   **11.29**
skeletal muscle vascular beds; although splanchnic and
cutaneous beds are constricted, overall peripheral resistance is reduced and diastolic pressure falls

    (d) **F**   Since diastolic pressure falls and systolic pressure rises,   **11.29**
mean pressure changes little, and reflex bradycardia is
not marked; thus, direct cardiac stimulation predominates

    (e) **T**   Dopamine has weak adrenoceptor actions and indirect   **11.29**
sympathomimetic effects, thus while increasing cardiac
output it also stimulates renal vascular dopamine receptors causing vasodilatation

Q30 In a conscious human subject intravenous injection of:

(a) α-methylnoradrenaline would cause an effect on diastolic blood pressure of similar magnitude to that seen with the same dose of noradrenaline

(b) metaraminol would cause a rise in total peripheral resistance

(c) phenylephrine may lead to atrial tachycardia

(d) methoxamine would cause bronchodilatation

(e) clonidine would cause bradycardia

Q31 In a conscious human subject, intravenous injection of isoprenaline would cause:

(a) a rise in diastolic blood pressure

(b) hypoglycaemia

(c) an increase in blood glycerol levels

(d) bronchodilatation

(e) tachycardia

Q32 In a conscious human subject, intravenous injection of:

(a) dobutamine would cause an increase in cardiac output

(b) propranolol would abolish tachycardia induced by a large dose of isoprenaline

(c) metaraminol would cause a fall in blood pressure

(d) salbutamol would cause bronchodilatation

(e) ephedrine would cause a rise in total peripheral resistance

A30 (a) **F** α-methylnoradrenaline is less potent than noradrenaline in stimulating α-adrenoceptors — it is this lesser potency that is thought to be responsible for its hypotensive action when it acts as a false transmitter *in vivo*   **11.30**

(b) **T** Metaraminol is a potent direct and indirect sympathomimetic that is used in hypotensive states to raise blood pressure   **11.31**

(c) **F** Phenylephrine is an α-adrenoceptor agonist; the pressor effect it causes results in a reflex bradycardia; this action may be employed to *suppress* atrial tachycardia   **11.31**

(d) **F** Methoxamine is a pure α-adrenoceptor agonist with no β-adrenoceptor agonism — it does possess some β-adrenoceptor antagonist effects   **11.31**

(e) **T** Due to decreased cardiac sympathetic and increased vagal drive, partly associated with a shift in the setting of the baroreflex   **11.32**

A31 (a) **F** Isoprenaline is almost devoid of α-adrenoceptor agonism, but causes a potent stimulation of β-adrenoceptors, leading to skeletal muscle vasodilatation, reduced total peripheral resistance and hence a fall in diastolic blood pressure   **11.32**

(b) **F** Isoprenaline stimulates hepatic β_2-adrenoceptors enhancing glycogenolysis and hence elevates blood glucose   **11.32**

(c) **T** Isoprenaline stimulates adipose tissue β (β_1?)-adrenoceptors enhancing lipolysis and hence elevates blood glycerol and free fatty acid levels   **11.32**

(d) **T** Isoprenaline stimulates bronchial β_2-adrenoceptors causing a reduction in smooth muscle tone   **11.32**

(e) **T** Isoprenaline stimulates cardiac β_1-adrenoceptors, an effect that is augmented by the fall in blood pressure, amplifying the tachycardia reflexively   **11.32**

A32 (a) **T** This effect is largely due to an inotropic action, and has been employed in the management of patients with heart failure   **11.33**

(b) **F** Although isoprenaline is a potent agonist at β_1-adrenoceptors it also stimulates β_2-adrenoceptors causing hypotension; the tachycardia is thus also contributed to by vagal withdrawal (reflex) and, therefore, would not be abolished by propranolol   **11.32**

(c) **F** Metaraminol is a potent indirect sympathomimetic with some direct effects; it is used to support the blood pressure in hypotensive states   **11.30**

(d) **T** Salbutamol is a relatively selective β_2-agonist that is used in the treatment of asthma   **11.34**

(e) **T** Ephedrine acts largely as an indirect sympathomimetic, and has been used to treat vascular collapse in allergic and anaphylactic states   **11.37**

Q33 Considering drugs with adrenoceptor antagonistic properties:

(a) phenoxybenzamine is a competitive antagonist of α-adrenoceptors
(b) phentolamine causes hypotension and tachycardia on intravenous administration
(c) chlorpromazine acts specifically on α-adrenoceptors
(d) ergotamine is routinely used in the treatment of hypertension
(e) propranolol acts at β_1- and β_2-adrenoceptors

Q34 In man, histamine:

(a) is largely stored in platelets
(b) injected intravenously causes cutaneous vasoconstriction
(c) causes increased formation of tissue fluid
(d) causes bronchodilatation
(e) causes increased secretion of gastric acid

Q35 In man, the effects of histamine on:

(a) gastric acid secretion are antagonized by H_2-receptor antagonists such as cimetidine
(b) bronchial smooth muscle are antagonized by sodium cromoglycate
(c) cutaneous blood vessels are antagonized by mepyramine acting at H_1 receptors
(d) capillary permeability are antagonized by corticosteroids
(e) gastric acid secretion are mimicked by ametazole

A33 (a) **F** Haloalkylamines alkylate α-adrenoceptors and thus their effect is non-competitive   **11.41**

(b) **T** Phentolamine has direct vasodilator effects as well as α-adrenoceptor antagonistic effects. The tachycardia is partly reflexively induced, but a component of this effect is not dependent on baroreceptor activity — it may be due to α_2-adrenoceptor antagonism   **11.42**

(c) **F** Although chlorpromazine is a potent α-adrenoceptor antagonist it antagonizes dopamine, 5HT, histamine and muscarinic receptors also   **15.5**

(d) **F** Although ergotamine is a potent α-adrenoceptor antagonist, it is also a partial agonist at these receptors and may cause an increase in peripheral resistance; it is used in the treatment of migraine   **11.44**

(e) **T** Propranolol has no specificity for the β-adrenoceptor subtypes   **11.46**

A34 (a) **F** Tissue stores of histamine are mostly in mast cells in which histamine is bound in large cytoplasmic granules, together with heparin and ATP   **12.5**

(b) **F** Histamine is a potent vasodilator; flushing of the face, neck, trunk and then limbs occurs   **12.7**

(c) **T** Arteriolar dilatation together with venoconstriction raises capillary hydrostatic pressure and hence promotes filtration; there may also be a direct effect on capillary permeability   **12.7**

(d) **F** Histamine is a potent bronchoconstrictor; this is a direct effect but there may also be a reflex component due to stimulation of afferent fibres. Asthmatics tend to be more sensitive to the bronchoconstrictor effects of histamine   **12.8**

(e) **T** Histamine is a potent stimulus for H^+ secretion by parietal cells, although its physiological role is not yet clear   **12.8**

A35 (a) **T** Cimetidine also inhibits the gastric acid secretory response to pentagastrin (suggesting the latter's effect is mediated through H_2 receptors). Drugs of this type are used in the therapy of peptic ulcer   **12.9**

(b) **F** Sodium cromoglycate inhibits the release of histamine from mast cells and thus is useful in the prophylactic treatment of hay fever, for example; it has no effect on bronchial H_2 receptors   **24.29**

(c) **T** Mepyramine has been routinely used in the treatment of allergies since 1944; it is a classical H_1 receptor antagonist (i.e. it has no effect on gastric acid secretion)   **12.11**

(d) **F** The usefulness of corticosteroids in treating immune reactions is due to inhibition of histamine release   **12.14**

(e) **T** Ametazole has about 2–5% of the potency of histamine on gastric acid secretion; it is used as an alternative to histamine in diagnostic tests of gastric secretory function   **12.9**

Q36 In man, serotonin (5-hydroxytryptamine (5HT)):

(a) is synthesized from the essential amino acid tryptophan

(b) biosynthesis is reduced by inhibitors of tryptophan hydroxylase

(c) is catabolized by monoamine oxidase

(d) biosynthesis is reflected in the urinary excretion of 5-hydroxyindole acetic acid (5HIAA)

(e) in the blood is largely contained in mast cells

Q37 In man, serotonin (5-hydroxytryptamine (5HT)):

(a) occurs in central neurones, particularly in the raphé nuclei

(b) occurs in the mucosa of the gastrointestinal tract

(c) causes inhibition of activity in the gastrointestinal tract

(d) causes cutaneous vasodilatation

(e) may be involved in haemostasis

A36 (a) **T** Tryptophan is hydroxylated to form 5-hydroxy-tryptophan and then decarboxylated to yield 5HT (serotonin); about 1% of dietary tryptophan is normally converted to serotonin 　　12.17

(b) **T** Tryptophan hydroxylase resembles tyrosine hydroxylase and also utilizes tetrahydropteridine as a cofactor; this enzyme is rate-limiting in the synthesis of serotonin 　　12.17

(c) **T** Monoamine oxidase acts on 5HT and other indolealkylamines to yield the corresponding aldehyde 　　12.17

(d) **F** Serotonin in the diet, mainly from fruits (bananas, strawberries, pineapples and tomatoes) contributes significantly to the urinary output of 5HIAA 　　12.17

(e) **F** The serotonin is mainly located in platelets, which may contain 1000 times the concentration found in the plasma; serotonin in platelets is taken up by them from the plasma, rather than synthesized *de novo* 　　12.17

A37 (a) **T** Cell bodies of neurones that synthesize 5HT are located mainly in the raphé nuclei; their axons project to the thalamus, caudate nucleus, limbic system, hypothalamus, midbrain and to the spinal cord (in bulbospinal pathways) 　　14.10

(b) **T** Most of the 5HT is found in the enterochromaffin cells in the mucosa — particularly in the gastric pylorus and upper part of the small intestine 　　12.19

(c) **F** Serotonin increases the tone and motility of most divisions of the gastrointestinal tract and enhances the peristaltic reflex; elevated 5HT levels in the blood, as seen in carcinoid syndrome, give rise to watery diarrhoea 　　12.19

(d) **F** 5HT is a potent vasoconstrictor, with a greater effect on venules than on arterioles. Thus blood accumulates in capillary beds and causes flushing 　　12.19

(e) **T** Damage to small blood vessles or endothelial cells causes platelet aggregation; release of 5HT from these facilitates platelet aggregation and also causes localized vasoconstriction 　　12.20

Q38 In man, prostaglandins:

    (a)   are synthesized from long-chain saturated fatty acids

    (b)   in the E and F series are largely synthesized in the lung

    (c)   are synthesized by a process which is inhibited by indomethacin

    (d)   in semen derive largely from the prostate glands

    (e)   are stored in large amounts in all tissues which synthesize them

Q39 In the normal human female, prostaglandin:

    (a) $F_{2\alpha}$ causes uterine contractions

    (b) E_2 causes a rise in blood pressure

    (c) E_2 stimulates gastric acid secretion

    (d) $F_{2\alpha}$ causes bronchoconstriction

    (e) A_2 causes diuresis

A38 (a) **F**   Prostaglandins are synthesized from the long-chain poly- **12.33**
unsaturated fatty acids, e.g. linoleic and arachidonic
acids, which are essential constituents of the diet

(b) **F**   Prostaglandins in the E and F series are catabolized   **12.34**
during passage through the lung; their pharmacological
activity is lost due largely to the action of the enzyme pro-
staglandin-15-dehydrogenase

(c) **T**   Indomethacin inhibits prostaglandin synthetase, the   **12.34**
enzyme that catalyses the first step in the conversion of
arachidonic acid to prostaglandins

(d) **F**   The main source of prostaglandins in semen are the   **12.35**
seminal vesicles and vesicular glands; semen contains
about 300 μg/ml prostaglandins

(e) **F**   Although some tissues store measurable amounts of pro- **12.35**
staglandins, it is likely that de-novo synthesis in response
to appropriate stimuli is the most important source of
physiologically active prostaglandins

A39 (a) **T** $PGF_{2\alpha}$ causes strong contractions of uterine smooth   **12.36**
muscle, and is used for inducing labour at term

(b) **F**   Prostaglandins of the E series cause arteriolar dilatation   **12.37**
and hence a fall in blood pressure; this effect may be
accompanied by an increase in heart rate and cardiac
output (due to reflex effects and/or direct central
nervous actions of prostaglandins)

(c) **F**   Prostaglandin E_2 inhibits gastric acid secretion; this may   **12.39**
explain why aspirin tends to cause gastric irritation (i.e.
inhibition of the modulatory effect of prostaglandin on
acid secretion)

(d) **T**   This is normally balanced by a dilator action of the PGEs;   **12.39**
it has been suggested that bronchospasm in asthma may
be due to imbalance between these two opposing effects

(e) **T**   Possibly due to a decreased medullary and increased   **12.39**
cortical blood flow causing increased glomerular filtra-
tion rate and decreased reabsorption

Cardiovascular System

Q40   In a healthy human heart:

(a)   the only connection between atrial and ventricular muscle is at the atrioventricular (AV) node

(b)   there is bicuspid valve between the right atrium and ventricle

(c)   the aortic valve is composed of papillary muscle

(d)   the pulmonary valve prevents regurgitation of blood into the right ventricle

(e)   oxygenated blood enters the left atrium from the lungs via the pulmonary artery

Q41   In the coronary circulation:

(a)   the coronary arteries arise at the aortic sinuses situated at the base of the aorta

(b)   the capillary:cardiac fibre ratio is similar to that of skeletal muscle

(c)   about 70% of the myocardial venous drainage enters the right atrium

(d)   communicating vessels between the coronary arteries and the left ventricle may either drain or supply the myocardium

(e)   the oxygen saturation of blood in the coronary sinus is similar to that in the inferior vena cava

Q42   Coronary blood flow:

(a)   amounts to approximately 10% of the cardiac output at rest

(b)   increases to meet the extra oxygen requirement of the heart in strenuous exercise

(c)   is reduced during hypoxia

(d)   is highest during systole and lowest during diastole

(e)   is reduced under conditions where the semilunar valves are incompetent

A40 (a) **T** Apart from this small connection, the atria are 22.2
separated from the ventricles by a fibrotendinous ring

(b) **F** On the right side the AV valve is tricuspid and on the left 22.2
side it is bicuspid

(c) **F** Papillary muscles are part of the myocardium (pillars of 22.2
muscle) which support the tendons (chordae tendinae)
attached to the flaps of the AV valves

(d) **T** This is a semilunar valve situated at the point where the 22.2
pulmonary artery leaves the right ventricle

(e) **F** The pulmonary artery takes deoxygenated blood to the 22.2
lungs; the pulmonary vein takes oxygenated blood from
the lungs to the heart

A41 (a) **T** The anterior sinus gives rise to the right coronary artery 22.3
and the left posterior sinus gives rise to the left coronary
artery

(b) **F** The ratio (which is about 9:5 at birth and 1:1 in adult life) 22.3
is approximately twice that of skeletal muscle

(c) **T** Most of this enters by the coronary sinus but some enters 22.3
from the anterior cardiac veins

(d) **T** The direction of flow in these vessels depends on the 22.4
pressure difference between the ventricles and the
vessels. During ventricular contraction flow can occur
from the chamber into the myocardium

(e) **F** The myocardial oxygen extraction is much higher than 22.4
that of any other tissue; hence the oxygen saturation of
coronary sinus blood is about 30–40% whereas vena
caval blood is about 70–80%

A42 (a) **F** The blood flow to the heart is about 75 ml/min/100 g, i.e. 22.4
about 4% of the cardiac output

(b) **T** Since the oxygen extraction by the coronary circulation 22.4
is normally so high, then any extra demand is largely met
by increased flow

(c) **F** Myocardial flow rapidly increases in hypoxia due to 22.4
reduced oxygen tension and to increased carbon dioxide
tension, or a fall in pH, together with accumulation of
adenosine

(d) **F** During systole there is mechanical compression of the 22.4
coronary vessels causing flow to fall to a low level;
during diastole the pressure in the aorta forces blood
into the non-compressed arteries at a high flow rate

(e) **T** Due to regurgitation of blood into the ventricles causing 22.5
aortic pressure to fall and ventricular pressure to rise

Q43 Cardiac muscle:

(a) is composed of multinucleate cells arranged as parallel fibres

(b) contains large oval-shaped mitochondria arranged in columns

(c) contains actin and myosin filaments which cross the intercalated discs

(d) has a well-developed system of transverse (T) tubules

(e) shows electrotonic coupling between cells

Q44 Considering the ventricular action potential:

(a) the rapid phase of depolarization is blocked by tetrodotoxin

(b) the plateau phase is due to a sustained increase in membrane sodium permeability

(c) repolarization is associated with an increase in membrane permeability to potassium

(d) the absolute refractory period lasts for about 10 ms

(e) the refractory period is almost as long as the muscle twitch which it elicits

Q45 Cardiac muscle contraction:

(a) develops greater tension when the initial fibre length is reduced

(b) occurs with a greater velocity of shortening when the load on the muscle is small

(c) develops variable force depending on the frequency of contractions

(d) reaches its peak at the end of the repolarization phase of the action potential

(e) occurs in a graded manner due to fibre recruitment

A43 (a) **F** In cardiac muscle there are uninucleate cells abutting at 22.10
the intercalated discs

(b) **T** These mitochondria (sarcosomes) are larger and more 22.11
numerous than those in skeletal muscle

(c) **F** The myofibrils of contiguous cardiac cells do not cross 22.11
the intercalated discs

(d) **T** In contrast to skeletal muscle, the T tubules of the 22.11
myocardium do not form regular diads or triads, but are
in close contact with the Z-lines of the myofibrils

(e) **T** The low resistance junctions between the cells (gap 22.11,
junctions and intercalated discs) permit passage of 22.13
action potentials from cell to cell in an all-or-nothing
manner

A44 (a) **T** This phase (O) is due to the membrane becoming 22.13
permeable to sodium and hence sodium moving into the
cell; tetrodotoxin blocks these fast sodium channels

(b) **F** The fast sodium channels rapidly close but there is then 22.11
a slow inward current, largely due to calcium ions,
which holds the membrane potential positive and
prevents repolarization

(c) **T** The inactivation of the slow inward current together 22.11
with increased potassium permeability (hence potas-
sium efflux) results in repolarization

(d) **F** Because of the plateau phase of the action potential, the 22.14
membrane is refractory to further stimuli for 200–300
ms (absolute values depend on the frequency of action
potential generation)

(e) **T** For this reason the cardiac tissue is protected from 22.13,
tetany 22.16

A45 (a) **F** There is a direct relationship between the tension 22.16
developed and initial (resting) fibre length — this is
known as the Frank-Starling relationship

(b) **T** The shortest latency and maximum velocity of shorten- 22.17,
ing (v_{max}) occur when the load is zero; the force-velocity 17.10
curve for cardiac muscle, like skeletal muscle, is
hyperbolic

(c) **T** In mammalian cardiac tissue this phenomenon is 22.17,
complex; it is probably a reflection of changes in 22.18
excitation-contraction coupling and calcium availability

(d) **F** The peak of contraction occurs towards the end of the 22.16
plateau phase; relaxation occurs during repolarization

(e) **F** Since cardiac muscle acts as a syncytium, it responds 22.16,
either as a whole or not at all 22.10

Q46 Cardiac excitation in the normal heart:

(a)   is initiated by spontaneous (pacemaker) activity in the sino-atrial (SA) node
(b)   is transmitted slowly (taking about 800 ms) through the atria to the atrioventricular (AV) node
(c)   is slowest in the middle portion of the AV node
(d)   is conducted down the interventricular septum in a single tract of conducting tissue — the bundle of His
(e)   spreads from the endocardial to the epicardial surface of the ventricle at a rate of about 0.3 m/s

Q47 With reference to the figure:

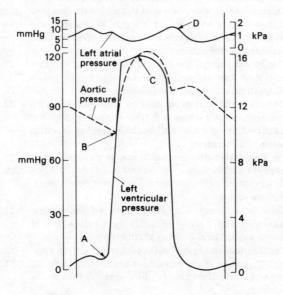

(Fig. 22.17)

(a)   the AV valves open at A
(b)   A–B represents the isovolumetric phase of ventricular contraction
(c)   the aortic valve closes at point C
(d)   ventricular filling begins at D
(e)   atrial systole begins at D

A46 (a) **T** Specialized cells in the SA and AV nodes show spontaneous activity; the slow phase of depolarization is thought to be due to a progressive fall in potassium conductance coupled to an increased slow inward current carried partly by calcium and partly by sodium — 22.19, 22.20

(b) **F** The conduction is fast (taking about 50 to 60 ms); some consider this is due to specialized conduction pathways, others that it occurs through normal atrial myocardium — 22.19

(c) **T** Slow conduction in this region (about 0.01 m/s) allows time for more complete emptying of the atria into the relaxed ventricles — 22.20

(d) **F** A single tract passes from the AV node through the fibrotendinous sheet between atria and ventricles but it then divides into left and right branches which run down each side of the interventricular septum — 22.19

(e) **T** Since the wall of the right ventricle is thinner than that of the left ventricle, the former may be completely depolarized whilst parts of the latter are still polarized — 22.20

A47 (a) **F** At the end of atrial systole, the relaxation of the atria together with the continued forward movement of blood into the ventricles produce reduced atrial pressure and the AV valves close — 22.22

(b) **T** During this phase, the AV valves are closed and the pressure generated is insufficient to overcome aortic pressure, hence there is no external shortening — 22.22, 22.23

(c) **F** Although left ventricular pressure only exceeds aortic pressure for about one third of systole, the momentum of the blood keeps it moving out of the ventricle (and thus keeps the valves open) until the end of systole when the back pressure in the aorta causes a reversed pressure gradient and the valves close — 22.23

(d) **T** At this point the AV valves open as ventricular pressure falls below that in the atria — 22.23

(e) **F** Point D marks the onset of diastole when both atria and ventricles are relaxed — 22.22

Q48 In normal healthy man at rest in the supine posture:

    (a)   left ventricular end systolic volume is about 20 ml

    (b)   the first heart sound coincides with the onset of ventricular systole

    (c)   cardiac output is approximately 75 ml/beat

    (d)   left ventricular end diastolic pressure is about 50 mmHg

    (e)   the second heart sound is caused by closure of the aortic and pulmonary valves

Q49 In an electrocardiogram recorded using bipolar limb leads in a healthy man of normal stature:

    (a)   atrial depolarization is recorded as an upward deflection in all three leads

    (b)   the beginning of ventricular depolarization is recorded as an upward deflection in lead I

    (c)   the R wave is smallest in lead III

    (d)   the process of ventricular depolarization lasts about 400 ms

    (e)   the T wave is recorded as a large downward deflection in lead II

A48 (a) **F** The end systolic volume is normally about 60–70 ml; this acts as a reserve volume   **22.24**

(b) **T** It is heard as a low-pitched 'lub' and is caused by closure of the mitral and tricuspid valves   **22.33**

(c) **F** This is the stroke volume; cardiac output is the product of stroke volume and heart rate (about 5 l/min)   **22.25**

(d) **F** In a healthy heart with efficient pumping, pressure falls close to zero in diastole   **22.24**

(e) **T** It is best heard at the level of the second intercostal space, just left of the sternum for the pulmonary component and just right of the sternum for the aortic component; it is higher pitched than the first sound (lub/dup)   **22.24**

A49 (a) **T** The vector of atrial depolarization (P wave) is orientated towards the left arm; it therefore produces an upward deflection in each of the limb leads, being largest in lead II and smallest in lead III   **22.29**

(b) **F** The onset of ventricular depolarization (Q wave) is not always seen — when visible it is only positive in lead III, since it marks septal depolarization travelling from left to right   **22.29**

(c) **T** It is reduced by a large downward wave (S) representing the late stage of ventricular depolarization; because of its direction it augments the R wave in leads I and II   **22.29**

(d) **F** The QRS complex normally has a duration of about 80 ms   **22.29**

(e) **F** The wave of repolarization travels in the opposite direction to the main vector of depolarization, i.e. away from the positive electrode; this produces a positive deflection (as does a wave of depolarization travelling towards the positive electrode)   **22.29**

Q50 Considering the diagrammatic ECG below:

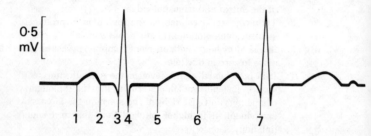

(a) the interval between 2 and 3 represents the time taken for electrical activity to conduct through the SA node
(b) the interval between 3 and 4 lasts for about 80 ms
(c) the interval between 3 and 7 can be used to calculate heart rate
(d) the interval between 2 and 3 represents atrial repolarization
(e) the interval between 5 and 6 represents ventricular repolarization

Q51 Cardiac sympathetic nerves:

(a) have preganglionic axons arising from the lumbar segments of the spinal cord
(b) have postganglionic axons in three bilateral nerve trunks
(c) innervate cardiac pacemaker and contractile tissue only
(d) contain both afferent and efferent axons
(e) have postganglionic cell bodies entirely within the stellate ganglion

A50 (a) **F** This interval represents the time when the atria are depolarized and the action potential has not reached the ventricles, i.e. conduction through the AV node   **22.29**

     (b) **T** This encompasses the QRS complex, i.e. ventricular depolarization   **22.29**

     (c) **T** This is the time taken for one complete cardiac cycle   **22.29**

     (d) **F** The atria are depolarized during this interval (see(a)) atrial repolarization is masked by the QRS complex   **22.29**

     (e) **T** The T wave is of longer duration than the QRS complex because repolarization does not occur synchronously   **22.28**

A51 (a) **F** Preganglionic cardiac sympathetic axons arise from the upper four thoracic segments   **22.33**

     (b) **T** The superior, middle and inferior cardiac nerves pass to the cardiac plexus which surrounds the origins of the great vessels   **22.33**

     (c) **F** The sympathetic nerves also innervate the conducting tissue — their stimulation enhances the slow component (phase 2) of the action potential   **22.35**

     (d) **T** The sympathetic afferents mostly convey the sensation of pain, although some are probably associated with volume receptors   **22.33**

     (e) **F** Some are in the stellate ganglion, but there are also some in the cervical sympathetic ganglia and the second, third and fourth thoracic sympathetic ganglia   **22.23**

Q52 Cardiac vagal nerve stimulation:

(a) reduces the frequency of SA pacemaker potentials

(b) increases the rate of repolarization in the SA nodal tissue

(c) reduces the refractory period in the SA and AV nodes

(d) has no effect on ventricular contractility

(e) may induce AV block

Q53 Cardiac sympathetic nerve stimulation:

(a) increases the rate of SA pacemaker discharge by acting on β_1-adrenoceptors

(b) produces a more forceful contraction when extracellular calcium is increased

(c) increases the frequency of contractions to a lesser extent when extracellular potassium is reduced than when it is normal

(d) increases left ventricular end systolic volume

(e) decreases cardiac efficiency

A52 (a) **T** The released acetylcholine increases membrane potassium permeability causing hyperpolarization and a reduced slope of phase 4 depolarization   22.34

(b) **T** Since repolarization is due to the outward movement of potassium, this is facilitated by the increased potassium permeability caused by acetylcholine   22.34

(c) **F** By some mechanism which is unclear, the effects of acetylcholine on the AV node are opposite to its effects on the SA node — in the former, the refractory period is increased   22.34

(d) **F** Although the parasympathetic innervation in the ventricular myocardium is sparse, vagal stimulation may produce a negative inotropic effect by: 22.34
   (i) reducing cardiac frequency
   (ii) reducing atrial contractions and hence ventricular filling
   (iii) inhibiting noradrenaline release

(e) **T** Conduction through the middle of the AV node is decremental, thus vagal stimulation may slow conduction sufficiently to cause action potential propagation to fail   22.34

A53 (a) **T** This effect is largely attributed to increased inward calcium flux   22.35

(b) **T** Up to a point, increasing extracellular calcium increases the force of contraction, but when external calcium levels are above those necessary to produce a maximal effect, β_1-adrenoceptor agonists cause no further inotropic effect   22.36

(c) **F** A reduction in extracellular potassium reduces the membrane permeability to potassium; reduced outward movement of potassium contributes to increasing the slope of the pacemaker potential   22.35

(d) **F** Sympathetic stimulation increases cardiac contractility and hence increases emptying and reduces the residual volume   22.36

(e) **T** Because of the increased force and rate of beating, myocardial oxygen consumption increases — this is proportionately greater than the increase in work done   22.37

Q54 In normal resting man, a bradycardia would be expected to occur following:

(a) increased carotid sinus pressure
(b) increased right atrial pressure
(c) application of pressure to the eyeball
(d) intravenous administration of a large dose of atropine
(e) inspiration

Q55 In the mammalian heart:

(a) increased extracellular potassium concentration reduces membrane resting potential towards threshold
(b) increased extracellular potassium concentration increases the membrane permeability to potassium
(c) hypokalaemia results in reduced ventricular action potential duration
(d) increased extracellular sodium concentration increases membrane resting potential
(e) increased extracellular calcium may counteract the effects of hyperkalaemia

A54 (a) **T**   Stretch receptors located in the carotid sinus and aortic   **22.38**
arch detect changes in transmural pressure; increased
distension increases afferent fibre discharge producing
increased vagal drive and decreased sympathetic
outflow

(b) **F**   Increased vena caval and right atrial pressures causes   **22.38**
an increase in heart rate (Bainbridge effect); there is
some debate as to whether this is a true reflex or not

(c) **T**   This is the vagal, oculocardiac, reflex due to stimulation   **22.39**
of sensory endings of orbital structures

(d) **F**   There is normally a resting discharge in cardiac vagal   **22.37**
and sympathetic efferent fibres; inhibition of parasym-
pathetic tone (with atropine) therefore increases the
heart rate

(e) **F**   During inspiration impulses from lung stretch receptors   **22.39**
travel via vagal afferents to cause decreased efferent
vagal discharge and hence heart rate increases

A55 (a) **T**   This effect would be predicted from the Nernst equation   **22.43**
and would increase excitability, i.e. increase SA node
discharge (but see (b))

(b) **T**   This paradoxical effect reduces the slope of the   **22.43**
pacemaker potential, tending to decrease SA node
discharge rate. The combination of the two above effects
means that heart rate may increase or decrease during hyperkalaemia, depending on which effect
predominates

(c) **F**   A reduction in extracellular potassium concentration   **22.44**
reduces membrane permeability to potassium with the
result that membrane potential falls, the slope of the
pacemaker potential increases (causing increased
excitability) and action potential duration increases

(d) **F**   The membrane potential is largely due to the disposition   **22.44**
of potassium; increased extracellular sodium is
excluded from cells by the sodium pump

(e) **T**   Due to the membrane stabilizing action of calcium, the   **22.43**
decrease. in membrane potential and increased
potassium permeability are offset. In addition, the
increased calcium gradient facilitates more inward
movement of calcium for contraction

Q56 Atrial:

(a) tachycardia is always associated with disordered ventricular rhythm

(b) fibrillation may predispose to embolus formation

(c) flutter may be abolished by application of a direct current shock at any stage in the ECG

(d) fibrillation may be reversed by application of pressure to the carotid sinus

(e) flutter is common in hypothyroid states

Q57 In the class of drugs possessing antiarrhythmic activity:

(a) quinidine acts by blocking calcium channels

(b) lignocaine may be effective in the treatment of atrial fibrillation

(c) propranolol is effective in the treatment of arrhythmias produced by overdosage with cardiac glycosides

(d) verapamil may be beneficial in the treatment of AV block

(e) amiodarone acts by prolonging the refractory period of cardiac muscle cells

A56 (a) **F** Paroxysmal tachycardia (100 to 180 beats/min) occurs at a rate which generally can be conducted through the AV node, giving rise to regular ventricular contractions. Flutter and fibrillation will, however, disturb the ventricular rhythm **22.49**

(b) **T** Particularly in atrial fibrillation, the absence of atrial contractions leads to stagnation of blood in the atrial appendages; the clots may then enter the circulation **22.50**

(c) **F** The shock must not be applied during the vulnerable period (just before the peak of the T wave) — this may lead to re-entrant dysrhythmias and ventricular fibrillation **22.51**

(d) **T** This procedure causes a reflex increase in vagal activity which may be sufficient to restore sinus rhythm **22.49**

(e) **F** Hyperthyroid states are often associated with atrial flutter. This may, in part, be due to interaction of thyroid hormones with the sympathetic nervous system **22.50, 19.20– 19.21**

A57 (a) **F** Quinidine exerts a membrane-stabilizing action by impairing sodium conductance **22.50, 22.51**

(b) **F** Although lignocaine resembles quinidine in most respects, an important difference is that the former has little effect on action potentials in atrial fibres **22.58**

(c) **T** The arrhythmogenic action of cardiac glycosides is partly due to increased sympathetic drive to the heart, hence the β-adrenoceptor antagonist is effective **22.59, 22.83**

(d) **F** Verapamil impedes calcium transport, and since AV conduction depends mainly on slow calcium-dependent potentials, verapamil will exacerbate the condition of AV block **22.61**

(e) **T** After chronic daily dosage there is a marked prolongation of action potential duration and refractory period in atrial and ventricular muscle cells. This effect is thought to contribute to the suppression of dysrhythmias **22.60**

Q58 Verapamil:

(a) causes coronary vasodilatation probably by blocking calcium movement into smooth muscle cells

(b) increases the slope of the pacemaker potential in the SA nodal tissue

(c) is a useful anti-arrhythymic agent in cases of recent myocardial infarction

(d) reduces myocardial contractility

(e) reduces myocardial oxygen demand

Q59 In the heart of a patient with angina pectoris:

(a) partial occlusion of a coronary artery by an atheromatous plaque results in elevated diastolic pressure beyond the lesion

(b) exercise may provoke an anginal attack due to a failure in the ability to increase oxygen extraction

(c) the endocardium is more vulnerable to ischaemia than the epicardium

(d) coronary blood flow may be improved by slowing the heart rate

(e) the direction of ventricular repolarization may be altered

A58   (a)   **T**   In smooth muscle, calcium stores are low and most of the   **22.7**
calcium required for contraction enters during the
action potential; by blocking this entry verapamil
prevents contraction of the smooth muscle

      (b)   **F**   The spontaneous phase of depolarization in pacemaker   **22.20**
tissue is partly dependent on an influx of calcium and is,
therefore, greatly depressed by verapamil

      (c)   **F**   Verapamil can be useful in some types of arrhythmia,   **22.61**
but because of the effect on myocardial contractility it is
contraindicated in cases of heart failure and myocardial
infarction where contractility is already reduced

      (d)   **T**   Calcium entry during the plateau phase of the cardiac   **22.13,**
action potential is important in excitation–contraction   **22.15**
coupling and is blocked by verapamil

      (e)   **T**   This is attributed to a reduced myocardial contractility   **22.67**
combined with reduced arterial pressure (i.e. afterload)

A59   (a)   **F**   It reduces the diastolic pressure (sometimes down to   **22.65**
about 25 mmHg) which, in combination with raised left
ventricular end diastolic pressure, reduces perfusion
pressure

      (b)   **F**   Normally the oxygen extraction from coronary blood is   **22.65**
near maximal; exercise is associated with increased
flow to meet the extra demand

      (c)   **T**   There is normally a greater arteriolar and precapillary   **22.65**
dilatation in the endocardial regions and a greater
number of functional capillaries to meet the extra
oxygen demand due to the high intramyocardial
pressure and tension. Since flow is normally similar in
epi- and endo-cardial regions, the endocardium is more
susceptible to inadequacy

      (d)   **T**   Since coronary flow occurs during diastole, the longer   **22.45,**
the period of diastole, the better the flow   **22.65**

      (e)   **T**   The result is often an inverted T wave; the change in the   **22.65**
direction of repolarization is due to subendocardial
hypoxia

Q60 Angina pectoris may be ameliorated by:

(a) an effect of glyceryl trinitrate on coronary arterial perfusion of ischaemic myocardium
(b) β-adrenoceptor antagonists, such as propranolol
(c) administration of hyperbaric oxygen
(d) oral administration of verapamil
(e) intravenous administration of the sympathomimetic amine dobutamine

Q61 In left ventricular cardiac failure:

(a) there is often peripheral vasodilatation
(b) salt and water retention is common
(c) there is a tendency toward oedema in the feet and legs when standing
(d) cardiac glycosides may produce a diuresis
(e) left ventricular end diastolic pressure is reduced

A60 (a) **F**   The beneficial effect of glyceryl trinitrate is probably through its effect on the systemic circulation (decreased arterial pressure reducing afterload, decreased venous return reducing preload); it has no direct effect on blood supply to the ischaemic region   **22.66, 22.68**

(b) **T**   These drugs are probably effective for a combination of reasons: **22.69**
    (i) reducing sympathoadrenal influences on the heart
    (ii) reducing arterial pressure (afterload)
    (iii) reducing heart rate

(c) **F**   Although this procedure can increase the amounts of oxygen dissolved in arterial blood, the oxygenation of haemoglobin is little affected since it is already near maximal. Excess oxygen may cause vasoconstriction and so aggravate the condition   **22.66**

(d) **T**   By inhibiting calcium transport, verapamil reduces excitation–contraction coupling and hence cardiac work   **22.67, Table 22.7**

(e) **T**   This drug has a greater inotropic than chronotropic effect and hence its effects on myocardial contractility may be beneficial   **22.67, 22.71**

A61 (a) **F**   The tendency for systemic blood pressure to fall is accompanied by a reflex increase in sympathetic tone, leading to peripheral vasoconstriction   **22.72**

(b) **T**   Reduction in renal blood flow and increased sympathetic drive (see (a)) stimulate renin release and hence activate the angiotensin-aldosterone system   **22.72, 22.74**

(c) **T**   Increased circulating volume (see (b)) and a reduction in plasma colloid pressure (due to the retained fluid diluting plasma proteins) causes increased tissue fluid formation   **22.73, 22.74**

(d) **T**   Their main effect is to increase cardiac contractility. As a result there is less reflex sympathetic tone and improved renal perfusion, leading to diuresis   **22.81**

(e) **F**   In the failing heart the stroke volume is reduced and hence diastolic volume and pressure are increased. Up to a point this may be beneficial since it increases fibre length and hence increases contractile force (Starling mechanism)   **22.74**

Q62 Cardiac glycosides:

(a) reduce the end systolic volume in the failing heart
(b) reduce myocardial oxygen consumption in the failing heart
(c) reduce myocardial oxygen consumption in the normal heart
(d) are more cardiotoxic when plasma potassium concentration is outside the normal range
(e) have a positive chronotropic effect on the failing heart

Q63 In the peripheral vasculature:

(a) large conducting arteries have the greatest wall thickness to lumen diameter ratio
(b) capillary blood flow is principally regulated by changes in diameter of arterioles and metarterioles
(c) the tunica media in the walls of veins forms valves
(d) dilatation of an AV anastomosis in the skin facilitates heat loss
(e) chronic overperfusion of a tissue reduces the density of the capillary microcirculation

A62 (a) **T** Their positive inotropic action results in a more efficient systolic emptying   **22.80, 22.81**

(b) **T** Since the volume of the heart is reduced by the glycosides (see (a)), then less tension needs to be developed to produce a given pressure (Laplace's law)   **22.81, 22.40**

(c) **F** In normal individuals, cardiac glycosides increase vascular resistance and hence increased myocardial wall tension needs to be developed, thus cardiac efficiency often is decreased   **22.81**

(d) **T** The explanation for the interaction between the glycosides and potassium is complex and ill-understood; it is most commonly seen with hypokalaemia   **22.83**

(e) **F** The cardiac glycosides have a negative chronotropic effect probably by: **22.81**
    (i)   reducing reflex sympathetic activity and
    (ii)   sensitizing the SA node to the effects of acetylcholine

A63 (a) **F** The conducting arteries have the most elastic tissue and are relatively less muscular; the small arteries (intermediate between distributing arteries and arterioles) are more muscular and have the greatest ratio of wall thickness to lumen diameter   **22.31**

(b) **T** At the transition between arteriole and capillary, the wall of the arteriole (metarteriole) may be relatively more muscular, forming a sphincter which can regulate flow   **23.1**

(c) **F** It is the tunica intima (endothelial lining) which is thrown into flaps forming valves   **23.3**

(d) **F** When the anastomotic channel is dilated, blood flows rapidly through it, in preference to the capillary bed, thus reducing the time and surface area available for heat loss   **23.3**

(e) **T** Underperfusion (ischaemia, hypoxia) stimulates the development of collateral circulations and vice versa   **23.4**

Q64 The arterial pulse contour:

(a) has a higher systolic peak when the elasticity of the large arteries is reduced

(b) has a lower systolic peak when the rate of ventricular systolic ejection is increased

(c) is a reflected pressure wave which travels at increasing velocity with decreasing vessel diameter

(d) has a steeper decline following the systolic peak when peripheral vascular resistance is low

(e) may be influenced by the haematocrit

Q65 Blood flow:

(a) is proportional to the length of the vessel

(b) is directly proportional to the square of the radius of the vessel

(c) becomes turbulent below a critical Reynolds number (about 1000)

(d) in skeletal muscle may increase during sympathetic stimulation

(e) in the pulmonary capillaries is reduced by low oxygen tension

Q66 Arterial baroreceptors:

(a) are primarily located in the carotid and aortic bodies

(b) have afferent nerves running in the IXth and Xth cranial nerves

(c) provide increased afferent input to the medullary cardiovascular centres in response to a fall in pressure

(d) have afferent nerves that synapse in the medullary reticular formation

(e) may respond less to an increase in pressure evoked by a vasoconstrictor agent than by an acute increase in plasma volume

A64 (a) **T** Normally the elastin fibres in the aorta stretch during ventricular systole and take up some of the kinetic energy of the blood — this serves to damp down the oscillations   **23.6, 23.7**

(b) **F** There is a viscous component in the elastic compliance of the large arteries which delays the rate at which they can stretch. Providing that ventricular filling has not been reduced, the effect of this is to reduce damping   **23.7**

(c) **T** Pulse pressure travels at about 3 to 5 m/s in the aorta, increasing to about 15 to 25 m/s in small arteries; this is because velocity of transmission is inversely proportional to compliance   **23.7**

(d) **T** The absolute diastolic blood pressure, and the rate at which it is reached, is largely determined by the resistance to flow during diastole   **23.7**

(e) **T** The viscosity of blood depends on the haematocrit and pressure is directly related to resistance to flow (dependent on viscosity). This can result in low blood pressure in anaemia and high blood pressure in polycythaemia   **23.7**

A65 (a) **F** Poiseuille was the first to demonstrate that the flow of simple fluids through rigid tubes is inversely proportional to the length of the tube   **23.8**

(b) **F** It is proportional to the fourth power of the radius, hence relatively small changes in vessel diameter can have profound effects on flow   **23.8**

(c) **F** Streamline flow becomes turbulent above the Reynolds number which is dependent on mean velocity × radius/viscosity   **23.8**

(d) **T** Skeletal muscle has a sympathetic cholinergic innervation, stimulation of which causes vasodilatation   **23.23**

(e) **T** This is opposite to the situation in skeletal muscle where hypoxia is a stimulus for dilatation, thus increasing flow   **23.21**

A66 (a) **F** Chemoreceptors are located in these bodies; the baroreceptors are in the walls of the aortic arch and carotid sinus   **24.9, 23.14**

(b) **T** The carotid sinus nerve enters the skull with the IXth cranial nerve and the aortic nerve (in man) is included in the vagus (Xth)   **23.15, 23.16**

(c) **F** A fall in pressure reduces discharge in the baroreceptor afferents, leading to reduced vagal tone and enhanced sympathetic outflow (due to spontaneous activity in medullary sympathetic neurones)   **23.15**

(d) **F** The nucleus of the tractus solitarius is the site where the primary afferents synapse; from there axons project to the medullary reticulum   **23.17**

(e) **T** Since they are stretch receptors, a constrictor agent that stiffens the arterial wall may limit their response   **23.16**

Q67 In normal, healthy man:

(a) central venous pressure is between 0 and 5 mmHg
(b) the a-wave on the venous pressure pulse coincides with ventricular systole
(c) about 70% of the total blood volume is in the venous segments of the circulation
(d) transition from the recumbent to the upright position is associated with a rise in total peripheral resistance
(e) blood volume falls during sleep

Q68 In normal man, cerebral blood flow:

(a) is about 300 to 350 ml/min
(b) is predominantly regulated by the sympathetic innervation of the cerebral blood vessels
(c) is influenced by changes in carbon dioxide tension to a greater extent than by changes in oxygen tension
(d) is lower in the cerebral white matter than in the hypothalamus
(e) is provided by the two external carotid arteries and the two vertebral arteries

A67 (a) T This can be taken as equivalent to right atrial   **23.11**
pressure — it would be elevated if right ventricular
output was impaired

(b) F The a-wave is caused by left atrial systole; the c-wave   **23.11**
coincides with the isometric phase of ventricular systole;
the v-wave occurs during diastolic filling of the atrium

(c) T The venous system has a large capacity, thus veno-   **23.12**
dilatation can cause a considerable reduction in central
venous pressure and hence cardiac filling pressure

(d) T Blood accumulates in the venous system and hence there   **23.22**
is a reduction in venous return, cardiac output, and
arterial blood pressure; this elicits a reflex tachycardia
and vasoconstriction

(e) F Blood pressure is low during sleep and there is an   **23.23**
increase in plasma volume due to decreased formation of
tissue fluid

A68 (a) F Cerebral blood flow is about 750 ml/min; consciousness   **23.23**
is lost if it falls below about 450 ml/min

(b) F The cerebral blood vessels have a relatively sparse   **23.14,**
innervation; present evidence indicates this innervation   **23.24**
is important in protecting against the effects of acute
elevations in blood pressure

(c) T Hypercapnia (increased P_{CO_2}) is a very powerful   **23.21**
stimulus for increased blood flow in the brain — this is
an important autoregulatory mechanism

(d) T The lateral nuclei of the hypothalamus, the posterior   **6.12**
pituitary, the pineal and the area postrema have a
particularly rich blood supply; the cerebral white matter
has a relatively poor supply

(e) F The internal carotid arteries anastomose with the   **6.12,**
vertebral arteries to form the circle of Willis which   **23.23**
supplies the brain

Q69 Pulmonary arterial blood pressure:

    (a)   is normally about 10 to 15 mmHg (mean)

    (b)   is reduced when the mitral valve is stenosed

    (c)   is increased under the influence of serotonin

    (d)   in diastole, is the same as right ventricular pressure

    (e)   when raised, may be detected as a louder than normal second heart sound

Q70 In essential hypertension in man:

    (a)   cardiac output is always above the normal range

    (b)   the reflex bradycardia in response to a rise in arterial pressure may be reduced

    (c)   medial hypertrophy is most common in the large conducting arteries

    (d)   intravenous administration of angiotensin II causes a greater pressor response than in normal man

    (e)   blockade of sympathoadrenal vasoconstrictor influences causes pressure to fall to a similar level as in normotensive man treated similarly

A69 (a) **T** Mean pulmonary arterial pressure is about 13 mmHg **23.25**
(20/5 to 49/15 mmHg; systolic/diastolic), i.e. about 80%
less than aortic pressure

(b) **F** Mitral stenosis will increase pulmonary venous **23.26**
pressure, which may then considerably increase
pulmonary arterial pressure

(c) **T** Pulmonary blood vessels are particularly sensitive to the **12.19**
constrictor action of serotonin which thus increases
pulmonary arterial, right heart and central venous
pressures

(d) **F** The two systolic pressures are the same, but during **22.24**
diastole pressure in the ventricle falls close to zero,
whereas that in the pulmonary artery is about 10
mmHg — due to the pulmonary vascular resistance

(e) **T** The second sound is due to closure of the aortic and **22.24**
pulmonary valves at the start of ventricular diastole; this
is accentuated if pressure in the aorta and/or pulmonary
artery is high

A70 (a) **F** In most cases it is peripheral resistance which is **23.30**
raised — cardiac output may even be below normal

(b) **T** This is a common finding in hypertension; the site of the **23.32**
disorder is not resolved, but one possibility is that vagal
efferent outflow is impaired secondary to abnormal
baroreceptor input

(c) **F** Hypertrophy occurs mostly in the small muscular **23.33**
arteries which provide a large component of vascular
resistance, hence the latter may be markedly elevated in
hypertension

(d) **T** An increased vascular reactivity to a variety of **23.31**
substances is often found; it is probably due to a
combination of medial hypertrophy and increased
sensitivity of the vessel walls

(e) **F** There may be a larger fall in blood pressure in response **23.31,**
to such treatment but nevertheless vascular resistance **23.32**
remains above normal

Q71 Secondary hypertension:

(a) due to excess mineralocorticoid secretion is initially associated with elevated cardiac output

(b) caused by renal disease is generally responsive to treatment with angiotensin-converting enzyme inhibitors

(c) may be produced by a persistent rise in intracranial pressure

(d) caused by phaeochromocytoma is most commonly characterized by a persistently elevated pressure

(e) caused by excessive intake of liquorice is associated with elevated plasma renin levels

Q72 In hypertensive man:

(a) treatment with a diuretic may reduce peripheral vascular resistance

(b) tolerance to ganglion blockade can be offset by administering a diuretic

(c) the adrenergic neurone blocker, guanethidine, is recommended if the hypertension is due to phaeochromocytoma

(d) intravenous administration of clonidine produces a prompt fall in blood pressure

(e) the hypotensive effect of clonidine is associated with a reflex tachycardia

A71 (a) **T** In mineralocorticoid hypertension there is an increased circulating fluid volume and cardiac output is high **23.28**

(b) **T** Renal disease generally results in underperfusion of the kidneys, which causes renin release. This promotes angiotensin II formation and hence aldosterone secretion; inhibition of angiotensin II formation is therefore beneficial **23.28**

(c) **T** This effect (Cushing's pressor phenomenon) is thought to be due to impaired perfusion of the medulla and to distortion of a neurone system in the pontomedullary tegmentum **23.30, 23.18**

(d) **F** In phaeochromocytoma episodic secretion of catecholamines by chromaffin tissues causes intermittent bouts of paroxysmal hypertension **23.27**

(e) **F** Liquorice has a mineralocorticoid-like action — the hypertension is, therefore, due to sodium and water retention leading to extracellular fluid volume expansion; as a result plasma renin levels are suppressed **23.26, 23.29**

A72 (a) **T** The mechanism for this is complex; initially there is a reduction in extracellular fluid volume and cardiac output, but secondarily pressure is maintained at the lower level with a lowered vascular resistance and normal cardiac output. Some diuretics may have direct vasodilator actions **23.40**

(b) **T** Ganglion blockade is often associated with fluid retention which reduces its effectiveness as antihypertensive therapy; this can be overcome by concurrent administration of a diuretic **23.42**

(c) **F** Guanethidine blocks neuronal uptake of catecholamines and hence produces a pre-junctional supersensitivity; it is, therefore, contraindicated in patients with phaeochromocytoma **23.43**

(d) **F** Clonidine initially causes a peripheral vasoconstriction with a rise in blood pressure; its antihypertensive action occurs later, due to central inhibition of sympathetic drive **23.47**

(e) **F** Clonidine causes a bradycardia — probably due to combined central inhibition of sympathetic drive and an increase in vagal tone **23.47**

Q73 In hypertensive man, propranolol:

    (a)   may produce muscle cramps

    (b)   may acutely result in an increase in vascular resistance

    (c)   is contraindicated in patients with a history of asthma

    (d)   is particularly advantageous if the patient has anginal symptoms

    (e)   predisposes to postural hypotension

Q74 Alpha adrenoceptor antagonists:

    (a)   inhibit the constrictor response to circulating noradrenaline more readily than the response to nerve stimulation

    (b)   cause a more profound lowering of blood pressure when given in combination with a β-adrenoceptor antagonist than when given alone

    (c)   are contraindicated in patients with a history of asthma

    (d)   may predispose to postural hypotension

    (e)   are equally beneficial in the treatment of essential hypertension and hypertension resulting from phaeochromocytoma

A73 (a) **T** This may be due to blockade of the β-adrenoceptor-mediated vasodilatation in skeletal muscle   **23.51**

(b) **T** There is an initial reduction in cardiac output (due to negative chronotropic and inotropic effects) and in response to this there is a reflex vasoconstriction   **23.51**

(c) **T** β_2-adrenoceptor blockade inhibits the sympathetically mediated bronchodilatation and hence predisposes to bronchospasm   **23.51**

(d) **T** The anti-anginal effects of β-adrenoceptor antagonists are probably due to a combination of reduced myocardial oxygen consumption, reduced afterload and lengthened diastole, resulting in increased coronary blood flow   **23.51, 22.69**

(e) **F** There is little, or no, loss of cardiovascular control during treatment with propranolol — indeed, sympathetic vasoconstriction is enhanced in the absence of β_2-adrenoceptor-mediated dilatation   **23.50**

A74 (a) **T** This is because the feedback effect of noradrenaline on to pre-junctional α-adrenoceptors (to inhibit transmitter release) is also blocked, thus more noradrenaline is released per impulse   **23.53**

(b) **T** Since transmitter release from cardiac sympathetic nerves is influenced by an α-adrenoceptor-mediated prejunctional inhibitory action, whereas postjunctional β-adrenoceptors mediate the response, α-adrenoceptor antagonism alone actually facilitates the cardiac involvement in the maintenance of blood pressure; addition of a β-adrenoceptor antagonist inhibits this effect   **23.53**

(c) **F** The increased transmitter release resulting from pre-junctional α-adrenoceptor antagonism leads to a greater bronchodilatation — hence these drugs may have potential use in the treatment of asthma   **24.31**

(d) **T** The reflex response is largely expressed through activation of postjunctional α-adrenoceptors; antagonism of these may cause incompetence of postural reflexes   **23.54**

(e) **F** α-adrenoceptor antagonists do not have a marked direct vasodilator action, but are effective in blocking the effects of circulating noradrenaline, hence they may be used to distinguish these forms of hypertension   **11.41**

Q75 In hypotensive shock:

    (a) intravenous noradrenaline is beneficial if the cause is haemorrhage

    (b) activation of the chemoreceptor reflex improves the circulation

    (c) peripheral vasodilators are beneficial if the cause is haemorrhage

    (d) adrenaline is particularly beneficial if the cause is anaphylaxis

    (e) part of the beneficial action of α-adrenoceptor antagonists is to inhibit the effects of excessive sympathetic stimulation on the heart

Q76 The development of an atherosclerotic lesion:

    (a) begins with the intra- and extra-cellular accumulation of lipid material in the intimal layer of the vessel

    (b) may be initiated by damage to the endothelium

    (c) progresses with the development of an amorphous lipid layer adjacent to the internal elastic lamina

    (d) may finally result in the formation of a three-layered fibrous plaque

    (e) principally occurs in small muscular arteries

A75 (a) **F** In haemorrhage there is already intense vasoconstric- **23.59**
tion, thus noradrenaline may worsen the situation by
reducing blood flow below a critical level

(b) **F** The chemoreceptor reflex produces bradycardia and **23.58,**
hypotension and hence would worsen the situation **23.18**

(c) **T** The beneficial action is through a combination of **23.60**
increasing perfusion to ischaemic tissue, relaxation of
pre-capillary sphincters increasing capillary perfusion
and decreasing peripheral resistance (i.e. afterload)

(d) **T** In this situation, adrenaline counteracts the bronchocon- **23.59,**
strictor as well as the vasodilator actions of the **13.24**
mediators

(e) **F** The reverse is true, since these drugs increase **23.60**
transmitter release (**23.53**) but do not affect the response
which is β-adrenoceptor-mediated

A76 (a) **T** The lipid material, rich in cholesterol esters, accu- **23.61**
mulates not only extracellularly but also within the
smooth muscle cells, transforming them to 'foam cells'

(b) **T** This facilitates access of plasma lipoproteins which **23.61**
promote proliferation of smooth muscle cells and
deposition of fibres and perifibrous lipid

(c) **T** This layer is made up largely of cholesterol and is, **23.62**
presumably, one of the reasons why hypercho-
lesterolaemia predisposes to atherosclerosis

(d) **F** The fibrous plaque has four layers — innermost fibrous **23.62**
layer packed with collagen; cellular layer with intra- and
extra-cellular lipid; inner and outer amorphous lipid
layers

(e) **F** It is the large conducting arteries which are prone to **23.61**
develop these lesions

Immunology and Haematology

Q77 In normal man:

(a) immunoglobulin G may occur in cerebrospinal fluid (CSF)

(b) specific G immunoglobulins are usually found in large amounts in plasma

(c) immunoglobulin M is predominantly intravascular

(d) immunoglobulin A probably functions to inactivate micro-organisms coming into contact with mucosal surfaces

(e) immunoglobulin E is found in high concentrations in the free form in plasma

Q78 In normal man:

(a) phagocytosis of antigens by reticuloendothelial cells prevents information about the antigens from reaching lymphocytes

(b) the immune responses may be inhibited by corticosteroids

(c) intravenous injection of a new antigen would tend to cause lymphocyte proliferation without formation of free antibodies

(d) excess amounts of humoral antibody may interfere with cell-mediated immune responses

(e) cyclophosphamide is a potent immunosuppressant

A77 (a) **T**   Immunoglobulin G is the smallest immunoglobulin and   **13.4**
normally occurs in CSF, saliva and tears (also it is the
only immunoglobin that normally crosses the placental
barrier)

   (b) **F**   Although G class immunoglobulins comprise 80% of the   **13.4**
total in plasma, a specific IgG is only formed in small
amounts after an initial exposure to antigen; large
amounts are formed and released on subsequent
exposures

   (c) **T**   This class has the highest molecular weight of the immu-   **13.5**
noglobulins and may be formed from large lymphocytes.
The proportion of IgM is highest after the first exposure
to antigen

   (d) **T**   This class is synthesized by plasma cells associated with   **13.5**
mucous membranes; deficiency of IgA is associated with
recurrent infections of the respiratory tract

   (e) **F**   Most IgE is bound to the membranes of basophils and   **13.5**
mast cells; reaction with antigen causes cell disruption
and release of contents — an effect responsible for certain hypersensitivity reactions

A78 (a) **F**   Although the antigens may not reach the lymphocytes   **13.10**
directly, information about them is passed on (possibly
by cell-to-cell contact or via messages released by the
macrophages)

   (b) **T**   Corticosteroids may cause involution of lymphoid tissue,   **13.13**
and inhibition of the recognition and proliferative
phases of the immune response

   (c) **F**   Intravenous injection of antigen favours a humoral   **13.10**
response, i.e. proliferation of B cells and release of specific IgM from large lymphocytes

   (d) **T**   If humoral antibody combines with all the antigenic   **13.11**
sites, then the antigen may be masked from the T cells
(such as may occur during the establishment of a
neoplasm)

   (e) **T**   Cyclophosphamide appears to act on quiescent and pro-   **13.29**
liferating lymphocytes

Q79 In the adult human:

(a) plasma albumin is synthesized in the liver
(b) elevated serum lactate dehydrogenase (LDH) activity is a good indicator of liver damage
(c) there are about 76 g of protein per litre of plasma
(d) plasma fibrinogen is synthesized in the liver
(e) an α_2 globulin, synthesized in the liver, is a substrate for renin

Q80 In the process of blood coagulation:

(a) prothrombin (II) is converted to thrombin (IIa) by platelet factor 3
(b) the role of thrombin is confined to the conversion of fibrinogen (I) to fibrin (Ia)
(c) the initiating stimulus activates factor XII
(d) the initiating stimulus may elevate plasma factor III levels
(e) defects in the final stages may be assessed by addition of thrombin to plasma

A79 (a) **T** Plasma albumin is synthesized in the liver and is largely broken down in the gut (after diffusion into the lumen); its half-life is about 15–20 days   **21.1**

(b) **F** Elevated LDH is seen with liver damage, myocardial infarction and skeletal muscle exertion. However, the isozymes can be distinguished, since those from heart and brain are more active than those from liver and skeletal muscle with α-hydroxybutyrate as substrate   **21.3**

(c) **T** Of this amount some 42–54 g/l is albumin and the rest globulins (α_1, α_2, β, γ)   **21.1**

(d) **T** As is the plasma albumin; thus liver damage can give rise to reduced levels of fibrinogen   **21.1**

(e) **T** Renin, a proteolytic enzyme, acts on angiotensinogen (an α_2-globulin) to form angiotensin I (a decapeptide)   **12.28**

A80 (a) **F** Prothrombin activation is effected by an enzyme complex formed by Xa and Va (requiring Ca^{2+}) and a phospholipid which may be platelet factor 3   **21.5**

(b) **F** Thrombin also facilitates the activation of V, (proaccelerin; Va facilitates the conversion of prothrombin to thrombin [see (a)]), of VIII (antihaemophilic globulin; VIIIa contributes to the activation of X) and XIII (fibrin stabilizing factor; XIIIa together with Ca^{2+} catalyses the conversion of fibrin (Ib) to cross-linked fibrin polymer)   **21.5**

(c) **T** Factor XII (Hageman factor) undergoes a conformational change which imparts enzymatic activity to it; XIIa converts plasma prekallikrein (Fletcher factor) to kallikrein which facilitates the conversion of XII to XIIa   **21.6**

(d) **T** If the initiating stimulus causes tissue damage, factor III (tissue thromboplastin; a lipoprotein released by tissue damage) levels in plasma may rise and together with factor VII and Ca^{2+}, cause activation of factor X   **21.5**

(e) **T** The clotting time after addition of thrombin to plasma is normally about 15 s; prolongation indicates deficiency of fibrinogen or the presence of inhibitors   **21.5**

Immunology and Haematology   75

Q81 Coagulation of the blood may be impaired:

(a) when factor VIII is deficient

(b) when factor IX is deficient

(c) when vitamin A is deficient

(d) immediately on administration of coumarin anti-coagulants

(e) by heparin which promotes inhibition of thrombin synthesis

Q82 Anticoagulant drugs:

(a) that are vitamin K antagonists have an action of rapid onset

(b) of the coumarin type are excreted readily in the urine

(c) of the coumarin type are antagonized by salicylates

(d) of the coumarin type are enhanced in their action by antibiotics

(e) of the coumarin type are antagonized by barbiturates

A81 (a) **T**   When inherited, this disorder constitutes haemophilia A   **21.7**
(classical haemophilia) and excessive bleeding may
result

(b) **T**   When inherited, this disorder constitutes haemophilia B   **21.7**
(Christmas disease); the two types of disorder (A and B)
are identical in inheritance and sequelae, and differ only
in specific replacement therapy

(c) **F**   Deficiency of vitamin K gives rise to reduced prothrom-   **21.9**
bin synthesis by the liver, and reduced plasma levels of
factors VII, IX and X resulting in prolongation of the one-
stage prothrombin time

(d) **F**   Vitamin K antagonists do not have an immediate anti-   **21.11**
coagulating effect; the latency depends on (primarily)
the rate of disappearance of vitamin K-dependent clotting factors

(e) **T**   Heparin acts at a large number of sites accelerating the   **21.15**
neutralization of factors IXa, Xa, XIIa and the inhibition
of thrombin synthesis

A82 (a) **F**   There is a latent period which depends on dose, potency,   **21.11**
endogenous vitamin K levels and particularly on the
rate of disappearance of vitamin-K-dependent clotting
factors

(b) **F**   These drugs bind to plasma proteins and so must be   **21.11**
metabolized in the liver before they can be excreted in
the urine. Hepatic or renal dysfunction, or drugs which
alter protein binding or metabolism by the liver, have a
marked influence on the activity of coumarin anti-
coagulants

(c) **F**   Salicylates prolong prothrombin time by antagonizing   **21.14**
the action of vitamin K; they also tend to cause gastric
bleeding and inhibition of platelet aggregation. These
effects enhance the action of coumarin anticoagulants

(d) **T**   Antibiotics (e.g. tetracyclines, streptomycin) reduce the   **21.14**
vitamin-K-synthesizing bacteria in the gut and so
decrease the availability of vitamin K

(e) **T**   Barbiturates stimulate the activity of hepatic microso-   **21.15**
mal enzyme systems and so increase the metabolism of
vitamin K antagonists

Q83 The anticoagulant heparin:

    (a)   is present in large amounts in blood platelets

    (b)   requires a plasma α_2-globulin cofactor for its activity

    (c)   has a hyperlipidaemic effect

    (d)   is routinely used in extracorporeal circulations

    (e)   is antagonized by basic substances such as protamine sulphate

Q84 Coagulation of the blood:

    (a)   is inhibited by plasmin, which is a proteolytic enzyme

    (b)   is promoted by urokinase

    (c)   is inhibited by ancrod, a thrombin-like enzyme

    (d)   is inhibited by aminocaproic acid

    (e)   may be promoted by aprotinin

A83 (a) **F** Heparin is concentrated in mast cells; it is released from the granules when the cells disrupt (as they do in anaphylactic shock) and inhibits coagulation   21.15

(b) **T** This is a proteinase inhibitor (known as antithrombin III), which functions as part of an intrinsic defence mechanism against thrombosis   21.15

(c) **F** Heparin has an anti-lipidaemic action due to liberation of a lipoprotein lipase from tissue into blood. Heparin has been used to treat hyperlipidaemia; this effect is seen with doses lower than those necessary for the anticoagulating effect   21.15

(d) **T** Its effect is rapid in onset but of short duration; its effect may be maintained by intravenous infusion. *In vivo*, its effect is rapidly lost due to plasma protein binding, uptake by mast cells, liver and kidney metabolism and urinary excretion   21.16

(e) **T** Basic substances that neutralize the acidic charges of heparin abolish its anticoagulant activity (probably by interfering with its binding to antithrombin III). Protamine sulphate is used to treat heparin overdosage and to terminate its action after extracorporeal vascular circuits have been used   21.16

A84 (a) **T** Plasmin is derived from plasminogen (a β_2 globulin); it hydrolyses lys-arg bonds at neutral pH. It converts fibrin polymer into soluble fragments and converts fibrinogen, prothrombin V and VIII into products which are not utilizable in the coagulation process   21.17

(b) **F** Urokinase, formed in the kidney, is a plasminogen activator (similar substances are found in other secretions) and hence promotes fibrinolysis   21.18

(c) **T** Ancrod produces microemboli which are rapidly eliminated from the circulation; the resultant hypofibrinogenaemia renders the blood incoagulable. It is used for the treatment of thrombotic disorders   21.18

(d) **F** It inhibits the formation of plasmin (and its action, in high doses). Aminocaproic acid is used for the treatment of excessive bleeding resulting from overactivity of the fibrinolytic system   21.19

(e) **T** Aprotinin (a peptide) is a competitive inhibitor of many of the enzymes of the coagulation and fibrinolytic systems; it is a potent inhibitor of plasmin and of the activation of plasminogen; it is used in the treatment of pathological fibrinolysis   21.20

Q85 Platelets (thrombocytes):

(a) contain large amounts of histamine
(b) promote haemostasis
(c) aggregate under the influence of ADP
(d) aggregate more rapidly in the presence of aspirin
(e) aggregate under the influence of serotonin (5HT)

Q86 Erythrocytes:

(a) contain haemoglobin at a concentration of about 5 mmol/l
(b) are produced at a greater rate when arterial P_{CO_2} is elevated
(c) synthesize haemoglobin from haem and four globin components
(d) have a lifespan of about 120 days
(e) have a relatively high rate of oxygen consumption

A85 (a) F   Platelets contain high concentrations of serotonin   **21.21**
(5HT — taken up from the plasma), ATP, platelet factor
3 precursor, platelet factor 4 (anti-heparin activity) and
an antiplasmin

(b) T   A low platelet count (thrombocytopenia) is charac-   **21.21**
terized by a prolonged bleeding time with a normal clotting time. Platelet aggregation is promoted by ADP, serotonin, catecholamines, thromboxane A_2, PGE_2, collagen
and thrombin, and is facilitated by platelet factor 3

(c) T   ADP probably acts by combining with a specific com-   **21.21**
ponent of the platelet membrane (von Willebrand factor)
and then complexing with Ca^{2+} to neutralize the platelet
surface charge which normally prevents platelets from
aggregating

(d) F   Aspirin (and other anti-inflammatory drugs) are potent   **21.22**
inhibitors of platelet aggregation; this effect is probably
due to inhibition of prostaglandin synthetase (PGE_2
stimulates aggregation) and ADP release from platelets

(e) T   Serotonin released from platelets probably acts on a   **21.22**
specific receptor to stimulate aggregation since the
effect is antagonized by 5HT blockers and by 5HT depletion with reserpine

A86 (a) T   This is close to the concentration at which crystallization   **21.25**
occurs; this mass of haemoglobin free in plasma would
markedly increase the viscosity and colloid osmotic pressure (by about 50 mmHg)

(b) F   Erythropoiesis is stimulated by hypoxia. A fall in tissue   **21.26**
oxygenation stimulates production and release of erythropoietin (largely from the kidney) which causes proliferation of erythroblasts and increased numbers of
reticulocytes and erythrocytes in blood

(c) F   The reticulocyte can make haem, globin and other com-   **21.25**
pounds from simple precursors; the erythrocyte has no
synthetic capacity

(d) T   Erythrocytes are normally replaced at a constant rate   **21.27**
(about 2×10^6 erythrocytes/s); old and damaged erythrocytes are removed from the circulation by cells of
the reticuloendothelial system. The protein goes into the
amino acid pool, the iron is re-utilized and the porphyrin
from haem is converted into bilirubin in the liver

(e) F   Erythrocyte oxygen consumption is very low and proba-   **21.43**
bly is a function of the amount of oxygen used in the
oxidation of haemoglobin to methaemoglobin; the metabolism of glucose by erythrocytes is entirely anaerobic

Q87 The biosynthesis of haemoglobin:

(a) involves the production of haem by erythroid cells
(b) involves the production of globin by erythroid cells
(c) may be impaired following chronic haemorrhage
(d) requires an intake of 0.5–2.0 g of iron per day
(e) always occurs at a rate determined by haem synthesis

Q88 In man, iron:

(a) absorption in the gut is increased at alkaline pH
(b) absorption occurs mainly in the distal duodenum
(c) is stored in the form of ferritin in liver, spleen and bone marrow
(d) absorption is maximal with a daily intake of about 200 mg
(e) absorption is limited by the rate of haemoglobin synthesis

A87 (a) **T** The starting point for haem synthesis is the condensation **21.28**
of glycine with succinyl coenzyme A under the influence
of δ aminolaevulinic acid synthetase (which occurs in
large amounts in erythroid cells and liver cells)

    (b) **T** In normal human adults about 88% of the haemoglobin **21.28**
consists of 2α and 2β-globin chains

    (c) **T** This may occur if the blood loss causes sufficient iron **21.31**
deficiency to impair erythropoiesis

    (d) **F** Absorption of 0.5–2 mg of iron/day is adequate for adult **21.32**
males and non-pregnant women; there is a need for
an additional amount (about 2.8 mg/day) throughout
pregnancy to allow for fetal and placental requirements
and blood loss in childbirth

    (e) **F** In iron deficiency or haemolytic anaemia the production **21.28**
of protoporphyrin by erythroid cells may exceed the rate
at which iron can be made available, so the erythrocytes
may contain large amounts of protoporphyrin

A88 (a) **F** Iron is absorbed mainly as the ferrous ion (Fe^{2+}) formed **21.33**
in the acid conditions of the stomach. The use of antacids
for ulcers that may be bleeding can give rise to iron-deficiency anaemia

    (b) **F** The ferrous ions are absorbed mainly in the proximal **21.33**
portion of the duodenum; addition of pancreatic secre-
tions impairs absorption, particularly due to formation
of insoluble salts (phosphate)

    (c) **T** The complex formed between apoferritin and iron-ferri- **21.33**
tin contains 20–24% of iron by weight. Ferritin stores in
liver, spleen and bone marrow contain 20–30% of the
total iron content of the body

    (d) **T** Larger doses saturate the uptake mechanism and pro- **21.34**
duce a mucosal block. In iron-deficiency anaemia a
maximal erythropoietic response is usually achieved
with 150–200 mg iron/day

    (e) **F** Excess iron intake causes accumulation of iron in the **21.36**
liver and pancreas which damages these organs; hence
there may be cirrhosis, pancreatic fibrosis and diabetes

Q89 In man:

(a) deficiency of vitamin B_{12} causes megaloblastic macrocytic anaemia

(b) deficiency of vitamin B_{12} may cause neuropathy

(c) vitamin B_{12} absorption may be impaired if gastric pH falls

(d) erythropoiesis would be impaired immediately following gastrectomy

(e) anaemia may result from chronic ileal disorder

Q90 In man:

(a) pernicious anaemia is effectively treated by eating raw liver

(b) folic acid deficiency may be combatted by eating liver

(c) folic acid deficiency may produce megaloblastic macrocytic anaemia

(d) pyridoxine deficiency may produce megaloblastic macrocytic anaemia

(e) chloramphenicol may produce aplastic anaemia

A89 (a) **T**   Vitamin B_{12} is required for the synthesis of DNA which   **21.36**
occurs at a high rate during erythropoiesis; deficiency
causes faulty cell division and maturation (macrocytes
are produced). The erythrocyte count and the total haemoglobin concentration are reduced, although the mean
amount of haemoglobin per erythrocyte is higher than
normal

  (b) **T**   Vitamin B_{12} deficiency impairs fatty acid metabolism   **21.37**
and thus may interfere with maintenance of myelin

  (c) **F**   Vitamin B_{12} is absorbed (about 1.0–1.5 μg/day) as a com-   **21.37**
plex with a glycoprotein (Castle's intrinsic factor)
secreted by parietal cells of the gastric mucosa. The
complex is absorbed by cells of the terminal ileum

  (d) **F**   Although gastrectomy impairs vitamin B_{12} absorption,   **21.37**
there are stores in the liver sufficient to last about 2
years

  (e) **T**   The vitamin B_{12}-glycoprotein complex is absorbed in the   **21.37**
terminal ileum — probably by an active, Ca^{2+}-depen-
dent process; thus ileitis can give rise to impaired vitamin B_{12} absorption and eventual vitamin-deficiency
anaemia

A90 (a) **F**   Although liver is a rich source of vitamin B_{12} the problem   **21.38**
here is an inability to absorb the vitamin. The most effec-
tive treatment is to give injections of hydroxocobalamin
(a pharmaceutical preparation of vitamin B_{12})

  (b) **T**   In addition to green plants (especially spinach) folic acid   **21.38**
levels are high in liver and kidney

  (c) **T**   Like vitamin B_{12}, folic acid is involved in DNA synthesis;   **21.38**
when deficient, cell division and maturation may be
impaired such that megaloblasts appear in erythropoietic tissues and macrocytes in the circulation.
Macrocytes have a shorter lifespan than erythrocytes,
and this exacerbates the problem

  (d) **F**   Pyridoxal phosphate acts as a coenzyme in the synthesis   **21.39**
of protoporphyrin. Deficiency of the enzyme leads to the
erythrocytes containing an excess of iron relative to protoporphyrin (the iron accumulates as siderotic granules)

  (e) **T**   Chloramphenicol in large doses may produce a mild and   **21.40**
reversible depression of bone marrow in all subjects;
some subjects may be highly sensitive and develop
severe bone marrow depression even with low doses

Q91 With reference to blood groups:

(a) individuals with type A blood could safely receive a transfusion of type AB blood

(b) individuals with type AB blood could safely receive a transfusion of type O plasma

(c) individuals with type B blood could, if necessary, receive a transfusion of type O blood

(d) a rhesus +ve mother may produce antibodies to the blood of her fetus if it is rhesus −ve

(e) the risk of complications in a rhesus-incompatible pregnancy (rh +ve fetus and rh −ve mother) is high

A91 (a) **F** Type A individuals have anti B iso-agglutinin in their plasma which would react with the B agglutinogen on the donor erythrocytes   **21.49**

(b) **F** Plasma from a type O donor contains both anti A and anti B iso-agglutinins which would react with the A and B agglutinogens on the recipient's erythrocytes   **21.49**

(c) **T** The donor cells contain no agglutinogens, thus as long as the volume transfused is small relative to the circulating blood volume and the donor plasma is diluted to prevent it agglutinating the recipient's erythrocytes this is an acceptable procedure   **21.49**

(d) **F** Only rhesus −ve individuals produce antibodies against the rhesus antigen   **21.49**

(e) **F** If it is the first pregnancy, the risk is minimal since the mother is not likely to have antibodies to the fetal blood. With repeated pregnancies, the likelihood that fetal erythrocytes have gained access to the maternal circulation during a previous parturition is increased   **21.50**

Respiratory System

Q92 In the respiratory tract:

(a)   the trachea is the only segment which contains cartilage

(b)   the submucosa of the trachea and main bronchi contains serous and mucous glands

(c)   the epithelium of the bronchioles contains a large
number of mucus-secreting goblet cells

(d)   the epithelium of the alveoli contains ciliated cells to
disperse foreign particles

(e)   gaseous exchange occurs in the alveoli

Q93 During quiet respiration (eupnoea) in a healthy human subject at rest:

(a)   the diaphragm contracts during inspiration

(b)   alveolar pressure is sub-atmospheric during expiration

(c)   the intrapleural pressure is sub-atmospheric throughout the respiratory cycle

(d)   the volume of gas exhaled per minute will be less than
12 l

(e)   dead space ventilation is approximately equal to
alveolar ventilation

Q94 In the pulmonary circulation of a healthy adult:

(a)   pulmonary systolic arterial pressure is approximately equal to that in the aorta

(b)   pulmonary capillary pressure is about 25 mmHg

(c)   vasoconstriction occurs in response to a fall in oxygen
tension in the inspired air

(d)   the bronchi are supplied with blood from a branch of
the pulmonary vein

(e)   the blood vessels are sympathetically innervated

A92 (a) **F** The walls of the trachea contain a series of incomplete rings of cartilage; the bronchi which arise from the trachea contain irregularly shaped pieces of cartilage — 24.1

(b) **T** The glandular secretions trap fine particles of dust and these are swept away by the ciliated epithelium — 24.1

(c) **F** In this segment there are only a few goblet cells. The 'Clara' cells, which secrete a protein-rich exudate, take over the role of the goblet, and other secretory cells — 24.1

(d) **F** Alveolar epithelium contains type I and II pneumocytes and phagocytic cells. The latter type engulf any foreign particles which reach the alveoli — 24.1

(e) **T** This process is facilitated by the large surface area of the alveoli. In man the total surface area is between 70 and 80 m^2 — 24.2

A93 (a) **T** Thereby increasing the volume of the thorax, decreasing intrapleural pressure, and causing lung expansion — 24.3

(b) **F** Alveolar pressure is sub-atmospheric during inspiration, hence air enters the lung — 24.3

(c) **T** However, the negative intrapleural pressure becomes more negative during inspiration than during expiration. The pressure increases above atmospheric pressure only during active expiration — 24.2

(d) **T** For most individuals minute ventilation is in the range 6–10 l; greater resting values indicate hyperventilation — 24.3

(e) **F** Dead space ventilation is less than alveolar ventilation at rest. Typically, dead space ventilation ranges from 1.5 to 2.7 l/min, whilst alveolar ventilation ranges from 5 to 8 l/min — 24.2

A94 (a) **F** Although average blood flows through the pulmonary and systemic circulations are approximately equal (there is a small physiological shunt due to bronchial and coronary circulations), the pulmonary circulation is a low-pressure system; systolic pressure is approximately 25 mmHg — 24.3

(b) **F** It is about 6–10 mmHg, i.e. less than the oncotic pressure of the plasma. Hence water in the alveoli is rapidly absorbed into the blood — 24.3

(c) **T** The physiological role of this response may be to direct blood towards a better ventilated portion of the lungs — 23.25, 24.18

(d) **F** The bronchial arteries arise from the aorta and supply the bronchi and other non-alveolar parts of the lungs — 24.3

(e) **T** Noradrenergic stimulation causes vasoconstriction. There are also cholinergic dilator nerves which may be vagal or sympathetic in origin — 23.25

Q95 During quiet breathing in normal man:

(a) diaphragm movement is responsible for about 70% of the volume of air inspired

(b) expiration is largely due to contraction of expiratory intercostal muscles

(c) the tidal volume is about 6–10 l/min

(d) the functional residual capacity is between 2 and 3 l

(e) the vertical movement of the central tendon of the diaphragm is about 1–2 cm

Q96 Concerning lung volumes and capacities:

(a) the total volume of both lungs is called the vital capacity

(b) the sum of the resting tidal volume and the inspiratory reserve volume is the inspiratory capacity

(c) the volume which may be forcibly exhaled in one second is greater than 70% of the vital capacity in a healthy adult

(d) the functional residual capacity can be measured with a spirometer

(e) the maximum ventilation volume is the functional residual capacity plus the inspiratory capacity

A95 (a) **T** However, this movement is not essential to breathing; in its absence auxiliary muscles may be used **24.3**

(b) **F** During quiet breathing expiration is largely passive due to elastic recoil of the lungs when the inspiratory muscles relax; expiratory muscles are more important during forced expiration **24.3**

(c) **F** The tidal volume is the volume breathed in and out in a single respiration — it amounts to about 500 ml at rest. With a respiratory rate of about 12 times/min this gives a *minute ventilation* of about 6 l **24.3**

(d) **T** This is the volume left in the lungs at the end of a quiet expiration **24.3**

(e) **T** This downward movement flattens the diaphragm, thus increasing the volume of the thorax, causing a fall in pressure and hence an inflow of air into the lungs to equalize the pressures. In deep breathing the downward movement may increase to about 7 cm **24.3**

A96 (a) **F** The total volume of both lungs is the total lung capacity; the vital capacity is the maximum volume of air that can be expelled from the lungs by forceful effort after a maximum inspiration **24.4**

(b) **T** A maximum inspiration starting from the normal expiratory position is the inspiratory capacity **24.4**

(c) **T** The ratio FEV_1/FVC is a useful index of airways obstruction. In the healthy adult it should be in excess of 75% **24.4**

(d) **F** The gas contained in the residual volume cannot be expelled into a spirometer. The functional residual capacity (expiratory reserve volume plus residual volume) is usually measured by nitrogen or helium wash-out **24.4**

(e) **F** The maximum ventilation volume is the greatest volume of air that can be breathed in a given time. Under standard conditions the subject breathes as rapidly and deeply as possible for 15 s, and the volumes are quoted in l/min **24.4**

Q97 Lung surfactant:

    (a)   is mainly produced by the type II pneumocytes in the alveolar epithelium

    (b)   decreases the surface tension of the alveolar lining during expiration

    (c)   release is stimulated by atropine

    (d)   production by mammalian fetus starts about half-way through gestation

    (e)   release is stimulated by β-adrenoceptor agonists

Q98 Lung surfactant:

    (a)   lowers surface tension and prevents collapse of the smaller alveoli

    (b)   increases alveolar surface tension as alveolar volume falls (during expiration)

    (c)   is deficient in the lungs of babies with respiratory distress syndrome of the newborn

    (d)   contains lecithins and sphingomyelin

    (e)   production is stimulated by glucocorticoids

A97 (a) **T** These cells synthesize and secrete this surface active **24.5**
agent which contains lecithin, phosphatidylethanol-
amines, sphingomyelins, lysolecithins, cholesterol, tri-
glycerides, carbohydrates and a specific protein

(b) **T** This is a special property of lung surfactant. During **24.5**
expiration, as the film of surfactant is compressed, so
the surface tension decreases and vice versa. Hence all
alveoli are adequately inflated despite their widely different sizes

(c) **F** Parasympathomimetics (e.g. pilocarpine) stimulate the **24.5**
release of surfactant

(d) **T** Its production increases until term. Deficient production **24.5**
of lung surfactant is responsible for the respiratory
distress syndrome of the newborn in which the lungs
cannot be held open after the first breath

(e) **T** These drugs are sometimes used to prevent an excessive **24.5**
decrease in the production of surfactant during open-
heart surgery when an artificial heart-lung system is
used

A98 (a) **T** In the absence of surfactant the smaller alveoli would **24.5**
collapse and empty into larger alveoli (due to the higher
surface tension in the smaller alveoli)

(b) **F** The particular property of surfactant is that surface ten- **24.5**
sion decreases with the area of the film; the converse is
also true. Thus surfactant stabilizes the alveoli with
changing volume and reduces the work of breathing

(c) **T** This deficiency prevents or impairs the retention of the **24.5**
functional residual capacity after the infant's first
breath. Instead, the alveoli collapse and must be opened
by positive pressure ventilation

(d) **T** There is somewhat more lecithin than sphingomyelin **24.5**
(the ratio should be greater than 1.5:1). Decrease of this
ratio indicates impaired surfactant function in babies

(e) **T** These may be used to enhance surfactant production **24.5**
when amniotic fluid samples indicate impairment of
fetal surfactant synthesis

Q99   In the respiratory system of a healthy human subject:

(a)   the pressure tending to inflate the lungs is the difference between atmospheric pressure and intrapleural pressure

(b)   the change in lung volume per unit change in transpulmonary pressure is termed the elastance

(c)   airways resistance equals transpulmonary pressure divided by flow

(d)   there is a straight line relationship between change in lung volume and change in intrapleural pressure during a single respiratory cycle

(e)   lung compliance changes directly with changes in initial alveolar volume

Q100   The work of breathing:

(a)   is decreased in disease states associated with reduced lung compliance

(b)   is increased by bronchoconstriction

(c)   increases with respiratory rate

(d)   in quiet respiration is greater during expiration than during inspiration

(e)   would increase in a healthy subject given a gas comprising 75% nitrogen, 20% oxygen and 5% carbon dioxide to breathe

A99 (a) **T** This is termed the transpulmonary pressure. At a con- **24.6**
stant atmospheric pressure, changes in transpulmonary
pressure are the same as changes in intrapleural pressure — the latter is rarely measured directly, but intra-
oesophageal pressure at the mid-oesophagus closely
matches it

(b) **F** This is the definition of compliance — the reciprocal of **24.6**
compliance is elastance. It is normally about 5 cm of
water/.l

(c) **F** Airways resistance is equal to trans-airway pressure **24.7**
divided by flow. Trans-airway pressure is the difference
between atmospheric pressure and alveolar pressure

(d) **F** This relationship forms a hysteresis loop due to frictional **24.6**
resistance to air movement and the properties of surfac-
tant

(e) **T** For this reason comparisons of compliance must always **24.6**
be related to lung volume so that an abnormality in the
quality of lung tissue or differences between individuals
can be distinguished from an abnormality or difference
in functional residual capacity

A100 (a) **F** Reduced lung compliance lessens the extent of lung **24.6**
expansion for a given inflation pressure, therefore
inspiration requires negative intrapleural pressures of
greater magnitude, more chest expansion and more
work

(b) **T** As above, greater chest expansion is required to over- **24.7**
come inspiratory resistance and active expiratory effort
is necessary to exhale; both processes increase the work
of breathing

(c) **T** Active inspiration occurs more frequently, hence work **24.6**
done per unit time is increased

(d) **F** In quiet breathing, inspiration is an active, and expira- **24.6**
tion a passive process, accomplished by elastic recoil of
lungs and thoracic wall

(e) **T** The increased inspired carbon dioxide level would raise **24.6,**
arterial carbon dioxide tension and cause stimulation of **24.8–**
the chemoreceptors; this would lead to a marked **24.10**
increase in rate and depth of breathing, and both would
necessitate increased work

Q101 In the medullary respiratory centre:

(a) inspiratory neurones show spontaneous activity when isolated from other neuronal inputs

(b) activity in the inspiratory neurones is reduced by lung inflation

(c) activity in the expiratory neurones inhibits the muscles concerned with inspiration

(d) activity in the inspiratory neurones increases, and activity in the expiratory neurones decreases, when CSF hydrogen ion concentration increases

(e) activity in the inspiratory neurones is increased by hypoxia in brain interstitial fluid

Q102 At the onset of inspiration:

(a) certain cell bodies in the medulla oblongata generate action potentials

(b) interneurons activated by inspiratory medullary cell bodies suppress expiratory neurone cell bodies in the medulla oblongata

(c) action potential frequency in phrenic nerve moto-neurones decreases

(d) all action potential traffic in respiratory tracts from the pons to the medulla oblongata ceases

(e) vagal afferents from lung stretch receptors become maximally excited

A101 (a) F   The respiratory centre becomes quiescent when isolated   **24.7**
from other neurones in the brain stem; it shows rhythmic
discharge only when influenced by action potentials
from non-respiratory systems

(b) T   This is known as the Hering-Breuer reflex. It is due to   **24.8**
afferent vagal discharge from lung stretch receptors

(c) T   The inspiratory and expiratory centres overlap and con-   **24.7**
nect with muscles concerned with inspiratory and
expiratory movements. Activity in one centre excites the
appropriate muscles and at the same time inhibits the
antagonists

(d) F   Increased cerebrospinal fluid hydrogen ion concentra-   **24.10**
tion increases activity in both inspiratory and expira-
tory neurones such that the rate and depth of breathing
is increased

(e) F   The only direct effect of oxygen lack by itself is to   **24.10**
depress neuronal activity due to decreased metabolism.
Oxygen lack does, however, enhance the effect of hydrogen ions on the respiratory centre

A102 (a) T   These are the so-called inspiratory neurones which acti-   **24.7**
vate phrenic nerve motoneurones, causing contraction
of the diaphragm

(b) T   This pathway abolishes expiratory drive during early   **24.7**
inspiration

(c) F   Phrenic nerve motoneurones *increase* their firing (see   **24.7**
(a)) and so activate inspiratory muscles

(d) F   Pontine neurones fire and contribute to suppression of   **24.8**
medullary expiratory neurones

(e) F   These nerves become progressively more excited   **24.8**
towards the end of inspiration

Q103 Peripheral chemoreceptors:

(a) are situated in the carotid sinus

(b) in the aortic bodies have afferent fibres which run in the glossopharyngeal nerve

(c) have a blood flow (relative to tissue mass) that is higher than for any other tissue in the body

(d) are sensitive to a 1% reduction in the oxygen in inspired air

(e) stimulated by excess carbon dioxide cause an increase in the activity of inspiratory and expiratory neurones in the medullary respiratory centre

Q104 The carotid bodies:

(a) contain cells which respond only to blood oxygen content

(b) have the highest blood flow, in terms of ml of blood per unit weight tissue, of any organ in the body

(c) are less sensitive to oxygen lack when blood carbon dioxide tension is raised above normal

(d) contain glomus cells which excite sensory neurones by cholinergic transmission

(e) may produce and secrete erythropoietin

Q105 The respiratory centre in the brain stem receives information from:

(a) the aortic and carotid bodies

(b) lung stretch receptors, via vagal afferents

(c) oxygen-sensitive chemoreceptors in the medulla oblongata

(d) receptors which respond to the hydrogen ion concentration in CSF

(e) mechanoreceptors of the larynx

A103 (a) **F** Baroreceptors are located in the carotid sinus; the **24.8**
chemoreceptors are in the carotid and aortic bodies

(b) **F** The afferent fibres from the aortic bodies run in the **24.8**
vagus; those from the carotid bodies are in the glossopharyngeal nerve

(c) **T** Their flow rate is about 0.04 ml/min and, in man, they **24.9**
weigh about 2 mg. Hence blood flow is about
2000 ml/min/100 g (compared to 420 ml/min/100 g in the
kidney)

(d) **F** They are sensitive to hypoxia but only when the normal **24.9**
oxygen percentage (21%) falls to below about 14%.

(e) **T** Both systems are activated and hence there is an **24.9**
increase in the rate and depth of breathing

A104 (a) **F** They contain cells which are sensitive to the partial pres- **24.8-9**
sure of oxygen. When this is normal but content (ml oxy-
gen/ml blood) is low (e.g. in anaemia) the carotid bodies
may not respond

(b) **T** They each weigh about 2 mg (in man). Their blood flow is **24.9**
about 0.04 ml/min, which is equivalent to 2 l/ min/100 g
— more than four times higher than kidney and forty
times higher than brain

(c) **F** Elevated carbon dioxide tension increases the carotid **24.9**
body response to hypoxaemia; the effect is multiplicative
rather than additive

(d) **F** The glomus cells are dopaminergic; they are modulated **24.9**
by afferent neurones via a cholinergic mechanism

(e) **T** Carotid body removal inhibits erythropoiesis; injection **24.9**
of a carotid body extract may then stimulate the process.
However, in man, the kidneys are probably a more
important source of erythropoietin

A105 (a) **T** These are the major peripheral chemoreceptors which **24.8**
respond to levels of hydrogen ions, carbon dioxide and
oxygen in arterial blood

(b) **T** These are activated during lung inflation, suppressing **24.8**
the drive to inspire further

(c) **F** The chemoreceptors in the central nervous system itself **24.10**
do not respond to oxygen, but they are stimulated
directly by increased hydrogen ion concentration, and
indirectly by carbon dioxide (see (d))

(d) **T** This is the major modality sensed by the central chemo- **24.10**
receptors. CSF pH may be decreased due to elevated car-
bon dioxide in blood diffusing into CSF and generating
hydrogen ions, but carbon dioxide does not stimulate
medullary chemoreceptors directly

(e) **T** These, when stimulated, activate the cough reflex **24.10**

Q106 The cough reflex:

(a) may be triggered by chemical stimulation of receptors in small airways

(b) is suppressed by expectorants

(c) is suppressed by codeine

(d) results in the generation of a positive intrapleural pressure

(e) is suppressed by dextromethorphan, a morphine derivative which is not addictive

Q107 In normal man at rest:

(a) the partial pressure of oxygen in alveolar air (at BTPS) is about 40 mmHg (5.3 kPa)

(b) the partial pressure of oxygen in pulmonary capillary blood is almost equal to that of alveolar air

(c) oxygen causes haemoglobin to oxidize to oxy-haemoglobin

(d) the affinity of a haemoglobin molecule for a fourth oxygen molecule is greater than its affinity for the first

(e) the oxygen saturation of haemoglobin in the pulmonary vein is about 97%

Q108 Gas exchange, between blood and alveolar air:

(a) is determined by the partial pressure gradient of the gas concerned

(b) is normally complete when the blood has passed half-way along a lung capillary

(c) is inhibited by oedema of the lung

(d) occurs more quickly for oxygen than for carbon dioxide

(e) is impaired in emphysema

A106 (a) **T** In addition to mechanoreceptors of the upper respiratory tract the small airways contain receptors sensitive to irritant chemicals — sulphur dioxide is a classical example   24.10

(b) **F** Expectorants increase the water content of airway mucous secretions making the cough more productive   24.11

(c) **T** Codeine and other opiates inhibit cough reflex pathways in the medulla oblongata   24.11, 16.6

(d) **T** The expiratory muscles contract against a closed glottis; intrapleural pressure rises markedly until the glottis is opened allowing 'explosive' exhalation   24.10

(e) **T** Dextromethorphan is a powerful antitussive which does not depress ventilation, cause tolerance or physical dependence   24.11

A107 (a) **F** The partial pressure of oxygen is about 100 mmHg and that of carbon dioxide about 40 mmHg   24.13

(b) **T** The barriers to diffusion of oxygen (surfactant, alveolar epithelium, capillary endothelium) constitute a distance of only about 0.2 μm hence alveolar air and capillary blood are almost in equilibrium   24.14

(c) **F** The reaction $Hb_4 + 4O_2 \rightleftharpoons Hb_4O_8$ is one of oxygenation not oxidation; the iron is present in the ferrous form in both states   24.14

(d) **T** This change in affinity is due to conformational changes in the subunits of the molecule. This effect, together with the combining ratio of 4 molecules of oxygen per molecule of haemoglobin results in a sigmoid relationship between Po_2 and oxygen saturation (oxygen dissociation curve)   24.14

(e) **T** With 100% saturation, 20.1 ml of oxygen combines with 14.6 g haemoglobin (present in 100 ml blood). 97% saturation in the pulmonary vein means that 19.5 ml of oxygen are combined with haemoglobin   24.15

A108 (a) **T** The gas partial pressure indicates the amount available for diffusion (i.e. that which is in, or can enter, solution); the blood–alveolar air partial pressure difference indicates the magnitude of the diffusion gradient   24.13

(b) **T** Indeed, one-third of the capillary transit time is normally adequate for complete equilibration for both O_2 and CO_2 24.13

(c) **T** When fluid is interposed between the capillary and the alveolus the path for diffusion is lengthened   24.14

(d) **F** Carbon dioxide is more soluble in water and diffuses more rapidly across the plasma membranes and therefore equilibration is more rapid although the gradient is less for CO_2 24.16

(e) **T** In emphysema the total surface area available for gas exchange is reduced   24.14

Q109 The oxyhaemoglobin dissociation curve (regression of percentage saturation of haemoglobin with oxygen (ordinate) against partial pressure of oxygen (abscissa)):

(a)   indicates about 95% saturation at an oxygen partial pressure of 100 mmHg (13.3 kPa)
(b)   is shifted to the left with decreasing pH
(c)   is shifted to the right in anaemic blood
(d)   is shifted to the right in the presence of carbon monoxide
(e)   is shifted to the left in blood from systemic capillaries

Q110 In mixed arterial blood:

(a)   the partial pressure of carbon dioxide is about 46 mmHg (6.1 kPa)
(b)   more carbon dioxide is carried per 100 ml when the partial pressure of oxygen is increased
(c)   there are normally about 42 ml of carbon dioxide per 100 ml of blood carried as bicarbonate
(d)   carbon dioxide (3 ml%) forms carbamino compounds with the plasma proteins
(e)   carbon dioxide is less soluble than oxygen

A109 (a) **T** Those factors which shift the curve (see (b)-(e)) have little effect on the degree of saturation at this level of oxygen tension because the relation forms a plateau in this range   **24.15, 24.9**

(b) **F** Hydrogen ions decrease the affinity of haemoglobin for oxygen, shifting the curve to the right   **24.15**

(c) **F** Since the ordinate shows the percent saturation, not the absolute amount per unit blood volume, the curve is unaltered   **24.15**

(d) **T** Even partial pressures as low as 0.5 mmHg carbon monoxide reduce the oxygen affinity of haemoglobin   **24.20**

(e) **F** There is a shift to the right in the capillaries (the Bohr effect). This is partly due to the elevated hydrogen ion concentration (see (b)) and partly due to the raised carbon dioxide tension   **24.15**

A110 (a) **F** The P_{CO_2} of arterial blood is about 40 mmHg. In resting tissues and in venous blood returning to the lungs the P_{CO_2} is about 46 mmHg   **24.17**

(b) **F** The carbon dioxide dissociation curve is moved to the right by an increase in oxygenation   **24.17**

(c) **T** 80 to 85% of the carbon dioxide in blood is carried as bicarbonate. This process depends on the ability of erythrocytes to form bicarbonate from the hydration of carbon dioxide under the influence of carbonic anhydrase   **24.17**

(d) **T** When haemoglobin is 100% oxygenated, all the combined carbon dioxide (i.e. excluding dissolved CO_2 and HCO_3^-) is in this form, whereas with haemoglobin free of oxygen, an additional 5 ml% of carbon dioxide is combined with the haemoglobin as carbaminohaemoglobin   **24.16**

(e) **F** The reverse is true and hence more carbon dioxide (3 ml%) than oxygen (0.3 ml%) is carried in simple solution, in spite of the difference in the partial pressures of the two gases   **24.16**

Q111 A patient has a pronounced transpulmonary vascular shunt through which a significant fraction of the cardiac output is perfusing alveoli which are not being ventilated. An arterial blood sample is taken and, on analysis, the following values are obtained; Pa_{CO_2} = 32 mmHg (4.3 kPa), Pa_{O_2} = 62 mmHg (8.3 kPa) and systemic arterial O_2 saturation = 89%:

(a) the Pa_{CO_2} is abnormally low because hyperventilation has occurred

(b) increasing the ventilation would restore the Pa_{O_2} and O_2 saturation to normal

(c) the oxygen dissociation curve for the patient's blood would be to the right of normal

(d) blood flow past the unventilated alveoli will be lower than that past the ventilated alveoli

(e) the patient would benefit from inhalation of an oxygen-enriched (i.e. > 20%) gas

Q112 Given the equation:

$$CO_2 + H_2O \rightleftharpoons H_2CO_3 \rightleftharpoons H^+ + HCO_3^-$$

it follows that, in a healthy adult:

(a) the concentration of hydrogen ions and bicarbonate ions in plasma are about equal

(b) production of appreciable amounts of lactic acid by muscle will increase carbon dioxide tension in blood

(c) hypoventilation will generate increased amounts of bicarbonate in the blood

(d) hyperventilation will reduce bicarbonate levels in the blood

(e) loss of hydrogen ions from plasma will lead to a decreased plasma carbon dioxide tension

A111 (a) **T** Hyperventilation, triggered by chemoreceptor reflexes, must have occurred for the Pa_{CO_2} to be subnormal (below 40 mmHg). The blood passing ventilated alveoli will lose much more carbon dioxide than normal and even addition of blood from unventilated alveoli with high Pa_{CO_2} does not elevate the value for mixed blood above normal   **24.18**

(b) **F** The blood passing the ventilated alveoli cannot collect more oxygen. Hyperventilation will not affect the oxygen uptake by the shunted blood, so its effect on the Pa_{O_2} and oxygen saturation of arterial blood will be negligible   **24.18**

(c) **F** The low carbon dioxide will have moved the curve to the left   **24.15**

(d) **T** Low Pa_{O_2} causes local vasoconstriction thus shunting blood to ventilated alveoli; prostaglandins, released by ventilatory stretching, may augment this effect by causing local vasodilatation near the ventilated alveoli   **24.18**

(e) **F** Oxygen saturation is as high as can be achieved under the conditions, therefore oxygen enrichment would not alter the hypoxaemia   **24.18**

A112 (a) **F** Plasma hydrogen ion concentration is about 40 nmol/l while bicarbonate is about 24 mmol/l. For electrochemical equilibrium the other cations (sodium, potassium, calcium, etc.) and anions (chloride, sulphate, phosphate, etc.) have to be included   **28.18**

(b) **F** The metabolic acid does give rise to increased amounts of carbon dioxide, but they do not stay in the blood, since the gas diffuses readily into the alveoli. Furthermore, the acidaemia stimulates ventilation thus blowing off carbon dioxide   **28.21**

(c) **T** Some bicarbonate will be generated acutely but, overall, hydrogen ion concentration rises (i.e. respiratory acidosis develops) because the ratio of carbon dioxide:bicarbonate is increased   **28.20**

(d) **T** Bicarbonate levels are reduced acutely but, overall, hydrogen ion concentration falls (i.e. respiratory alkalosis develops) because the ratio of carbon dioxide:bicarbonate is reduced   **28.20**

(e) **F** Loss of hydrogen ions (e.g. due to vomiting) produces a metabolic alkalosis which leads to a depression of ventilation and hence a rise in plasma carbon dioxide tension   **24.10, 28.20**

Q113 In man, hypoxia:

(a) developing at high altitude shifts the oxyhaemoglobin dissociation curve to the left

(b) is usually accompanied by Cheyne-Stokes breathing

(c) of the anaemic type is usually associated with an increased cardiac output

(d) of the stagnant type, due to heart failure, is often associated with an increased arteriovenous oxygen difference

(e) due to carbon monoxide poisoning is characterized by cyanosis

Q114 Analeptic drugs (respiratory stimulants):

(a) stimulate certain neurones in the medulla oblongata

(b) lower systemic arterial pressure

(c) can cause clonic convulsions

(d) increase the rate of breathing without affecting tidal volume

(e) are selective antagonists towards barbiturate-induced central nervous depression

A113 (a) **F**   Although the hyperventilation resulting from hypoxia   **24.20**
reduces blood carbon dioxide levels (which would shift
the curve to the left), elevated glycolysis in erythrocytes
(and other tissues) increases 2–3-diphosphoglycerate
levels which increases the delivery of oxygen to tissues
(i.e. shifts the curve to the right)

      (b) **F**   Although Cheyne-Stokes breathing (breaths separated   **24.19**
by apnoeic periods) occurs in some cases of hypoxia, it is
usually an ominous sign only associated with serious
respiratory centre depression

      (c) **F**   There is an increase in 2–3-diphosphoglycerate levels   **24.20**
(reducing the affinity of haemoglobin for oxygen) and a
redistribution of blood flow to perfuse essential tissues
but cardiac output is little affected until haemoglobin
falls below about 65% normal

      (d) **T**   Blood is redirected from skin, kidneys and splanchnic   **24.21**
beds to more 'essential' tissues. Erythrocyte 2–3-
diphosphoglycerate production is increased and so there
is a greater unloading of oxygen from haemoglobin in the
perfused tissues resulting in an increased arteriovenous
oxygen difference

      (e) **F**   Hypoxia is associated with cyanosis (blue colouration   **24.20**
due to high levels of deoxygenated haemoglobin) but car-
boxyhaemoglobin is bright red and this colour is visible
in skin, nail beds and mucous membranes

A114 (a) **T**   They stimulate certain neurones in the respiratory cen-   **24.22**
tre of the medulla, thereby increasing ventilation

      (b) **F**   They elevate systemic arterial pressure via central   **24.22**
actions on the vasomotor centre

      (c) **T**   This occurs, usually at higher doses than the brain stem   **24.22**
effects, due to stimulation of the motor cortex

      (d) **F**   Both rate and tidal volume increase; such drugs may be   **24.22**
useful in the treatment of hypercapnia combined with
hypoxaemia

      (e) **F**   This was formerly thought to be true for bemegride, but   **24.23**
it is now established that analeptics antagonize any
respiratory depressant

Q115 Elevation of airway resistance (for instance by bronchocon-striction) would:

(a) decrease the volume of air which could be exhaled forcibly in one second (FEV_1)
(b) decrease the work of breathing
(c) reduce the functional residual capacity (FRC)
(d) reduce peak expiratory flow
(e) increase the bronchial breath sounds

Q116 Salbutamol:

(a) is a β_1-selective adrenoceptor agonist
(b) acts on the lung only when administered by inhalation
(c) is less selective towards bronchodilator β-adrenocep-tors than is isoprenaline
(d) reduces the FEV_1 in asthmatics
(e) may cause vasodilatation in skeletal muscle

Q117 An attack of bronchoconstriction would be expected to be relieved by:

(a) inhalation of salbutamol
(b) inhalation of disodium cromoglycate
(c) intravenous aminophylline
(d) propranolol
(e) inhalation of beclomethasone

A115 (a) **T** The flow attained in response to a given transpulmonary pressure is limited by the airway resistance (c.f. Poiseuille's Law), hence exhaled volume per unit time falls — 24.24

(b) **F** To maintain normal ventilation, greater inspiratory and expiratory pressures would be needed, hence the work of breathing would rise — 24.24

(c) **F** Airway resistance decreases with increasing lung volume; bronchoconstriction therefore causes the subconscious adaptation of breathing with increased FRC so as to minimize the work of breathing — 24.24

(d) **T** For the reasons given above, both FEV_1 and peak expiratory flow are reduced — 24.24

(e) **T** These may be dramatically audible without a stethoscope — the characteristic wheezing of asthma — 24.24

A116 (a) **F** Salbutamol is a β-adrenoceptor agonist which shows selectivity towards β_2-adrenoceptors — 24.26

(b) **F** Although salbutamol is frequently given by inhalation it can be given by intramuscular or subcutaneous injection and is even active after oral administration — 11.34

(c) **F** Isoprenaline shows no selectivity between β_1 and β_2 subtypes of adrenoceptor, hence salbutamol is now preferred because of its less marked effects on the heart (β_1-receptor mediated) — 24.26

(d) **F** The bronchodilatation produced by salbutamol causes an increase in FEV_1 — 24.24, 24.26

(e) **T** The vasodilator adrenoceptors in skeletal muscle arterioles are of the β_2 sub-type — 11.29

A117 (a) **T** Salbutamol is a selective β_2-adrenoceptor agonist; it would relax bronchial smooth muscle decreasing airway resistance — 24.26

(b) **F** Although disodium cromoglycate is effective against allergic asthma, it must be used prophylactically and is ineffective once an attack has begun — 24.29

(c) **T** Aminophylline contains the xanthine, theophylline, which causes bronchodilatation probably via release of noradrenaline and stimulation of pulmonary β_2-adrenoceptors; it is usually given intravenously — 24.28

(d) **F** Propranolol would block pulmonary β-adrenoceptors and may exacerbate bronchoconstriction. Its use for other conditions (e.g. hypertension) is, therefore, contraindicated in asthma — 24.26

(e) **T** Beclomethasone is an anti-inflammatory steroid. It reduces release of bronchoconstrictor autacoids and ameliorates mucosal oedema of the airways — 24.29

Q118 Sodium cromoglycate:

- (a) acts directly on bronchial smooth muscle to induce relaxation
- (b) is most effective in asthma when administered by inhalation
- (c) reduces antigen-induced release of histamine from sensitized human lung tissue
- (d) inhibits the binding of IgE antibodies to mast cells
- (e) may act to inhibit antigen-induced increases in mast cell calcium permeability

A118 (a) **F** Sodium cromoglycate has no demonstrable direct effects on the tone or contractility of bronchial smooth muscle 24.29

  (b) **T** The absorption from other routes is poor and plasma half-life very short 24.30

  (c) **T** This is demonstrable by experiment; the release of SRS-A (slow reacting substance — anaphylaxis) is reduced concurrently 24.30

  (d) **F** The drug is without demonstrable effect on cell fixation of the antibodies which mediate asthmatic bronchoconstriction 24.30

  (e) **T** This is currently thought to be one of the most likely mechanisms of action 24.30

Locomotor System

Q119 In the skeletal muscle cell:

   (a)   the A bands demarcate the region of overlap of actin
         and myosin filaments
   (b)   the T-tubules run closest to the M line
   (c)   actin-to-myosin cross bridges are present only in the
         H zone
   (d)   actin has a larger molecular weight than myosin
   (e)   there are many nuclei

Q120 In the skeletal muscle cell:

   (a)   propagation of an action potential initiates con-
         traction
   (b)   the action potential causes depolarization to be
         conducted through the T-tubules
   (c)   the T-tubules release the majority of the free
         intracellular calcium ions during contraction
   (d)   calcium ions bind to the troponin-tropomyosin com-
         plex during contraction
   (e)   myosin hydrolyses ATP during contraction

Q121 In skeletal muscle, calcium ions:

   (a)   bind to smooth endoplasmic reticulum at the onset of
         contraction
   (b)   show increased affinity of binding to smooth endo-
         plasmic reticulum when ATP is present
   (c)   compete with magnesium ions for binding to troponin-
         tropomyosin
   (d)   may be taken up by mitochondria during relaxation
   (e)   increase progressively in concentration in the sar-
         coplasm during tetanic contraction

A119 (a) **T** The overlap zone has the greatest density of microfilaments and shows up as the darkest striation — 17.2

(b) **F** The T-tubules circumscribe the Z-line — 17.2

(c) **F** Cross-bridges are absent from the H zone but present throughout the remainder of the A band — 17.2, 17.3

(d) **F** Myosin, comprising the thick filaments, has a molecular weight of about 470 000. Actin, forming the thin filaments, has a molecular weight of about 46 000 — 17.3

(e) **T** Each cell is multinucleate — 17.1

A120 (a) **T** Excitation from motor end plates generates action potentials which spread through the cells triggering the processes described below — 17.4

(b) **T** The T-tubules are contiguous with the sarcolemma thereby giving electrical continuity with the interior of the cell where the contractile apparatus is situated — 17.5

(c) **F** The T-tubules release small amounts of so-called 'trigger Ca^{2+}'. This causes release of much larger amounts of calcium from the sarcoplasmic reticulum — 17.5

(d) **T** This removes the inhibitory influence of troponin-tropomyosin on cross-bridge formation thereby enabling contraction — 17.5

(e) **T** This permits cross-bridges to form and energizes the sliding of the filaments — 17.6

A121 (a) **F** The smooth endoplasmic reticulum *releases* Ca^{2+} into the sarcoplasm at the onset of contraction — this process is triggered by Ca^{2+} released from the T-tubules. Binding of Ca^{2+} by smooth endoplasmic reticulum is inhibited (see (b)) until it occurs to promote relaxation — 17.6

(b) **T** The hydrolysis of ATP by smooth endoplasmic reticulum-ATPase promotes binding of Ca^{2+} and ATP also increases the affinity for Ca^{2+} — 17.6

(c) **T** There is stoichiometric competition between the two cations. Ca^{2+} binding removes troponin-tropomyosin from the filaments to promote sliding; magnesium has the opposite effect — 17.6

(d) **T** Muscle mitochondria have a large capacity to store calcium; they remove it from sarcoplasm more slowly than does the smooth endoplasmic reticulum, but the mitochondria do participate in relaxation — 17.6

(e) **T** With each action potential the concentration of free calcium increases to build up contractile force — 17.8

Q122 Skeletal muscle contraction:

(a) in which the muscle shortens under constant load is said to be isotonic

(b) in which tension is developed at fixed length is said to be isometric

(c) shows the greatest mechanical efficiency when the load presented to the muscle is about one tenth of the maximum that can be moved

(d) may be increased in strength, for a whole muscle, by progressive recruitment of motor units

(e) may be increased in strength, for a single motor unit, by increasing stimulation frequency

Q123 In skeletal muscle:

(a) red fibres contain more myoglobin than white fibres

(b) white fibres contain the most sparse smooth endoplasmic reticulum (SER) of the three fibre types

(c) red fibres fatigue more quickly than white fibres

(d) white fibres have the highest capacity for anaerobic glucose metabolism

(e) red fibres are the dominant type in the diaphragm

Q124 In skeletal muscle:

(a) red muscle fibres are slow-contracting

(b) flexor muscles contain predominantly slow-contracting fibres

(c) the myosin ATPase hydrolyses ATP more rapidly in fast than in slow fibres

(d) the sarcoplasmic reticulum is more extensive in fast than in slow fibres

(e) fast and slow fibres may each have a single motor end plate

A122 (a) **T** This occurs in walking or lifting **17.8**

(b) **T** This occurs when stationary posture is maintained against the force of gravity **17.8**

(c) **F** Efficiency (in terms of power output) is maximal when load and speed of shortening are about ⅓ maximal **17.10**

(d) **T** Recruitment of motor units of increasing size contributes to the graded contraction of the whole muscle **17.19**

(e) **T** Motoneurone firing frequency is in the range 5 to 100 Hz. As frequency increases, so a staircase effect develops into fused tetany. The maximum tetanic force is considerably greater than that generated by individual twitches **17.19**

A123 (a) **T** This is the basis on which they are so classified; intermediate fibres are also high in myoglobin **17.11**

(b) **F** Intermediate fibres contain the most sparse SER. White and red fibres have well-developed SER which sequesters Ca^{2+} rapidly, giving a fast twitch response **17.11**

(c) **F** White fibres fatigue more quickly than red, hence white fibres are adapted for rapid, brief, intermittent activity, whilst red fibres are more suited to sustained phasic activity such as in breathing or flight **17.11, 17.12**

(d) **T** Thus their anaerobic glycolytic metabolism enables fast ATP production and the ensuing oxygen debt may be repaid during the periods of inactivity undergone by this type of muscle **17.11**

(e) **T** See (c); this type of muscle is suited to ventilatory activity. The rat diaphragm contains 60% red, 20% intermediate and 20% white fibres **17.11**

A124 (a) **F** Intermediate fibres are slow; both red and white are fast-contracting **17.12, Table 17.2**

(b) **F** Mammalian flexor muscles contain fast-contracting fibres **17.12**

(c) **T** Hydrolysis of ATP by myosin ATPase is the rate-limiting step in contraction; it limits the maximum rate at which the interdigitated thick and thin filaments can slide **17.12**

(d) **T** There is about twice as much sarcoplasmic reticulum in fast than in slow fibres, and it makes more frequent contacts with T-tubules; the rate of Ca^{2+} sequestration is faster in fast fibres, thus relaxation (as well as contraction) is more rapid **17.12**

(e) **T** Such fibres are said to be focally innervated (see **Fig. 17.14**). A very small number of mammalian muscles differ from this pattern in that they receive a multiple innervation **17.19**

Q125 In skeletal muscle:

(a) tetrodotoxin blocks membrane calcium channels

(b) thiocyanate ions lower the threshold for mechanical activation

(c) caffeine potentiates contraction by inhibition of phosphodiesterase

(d) β_2-selective adrenoceptor agonists increase twitch tension in fast contracting fibres

(e) excessive circulating thyroid hormones cause tremor

Q126 A typical mammalian motoneurone:

(a) innervates only one skeletal muscle cell

(b) has a myelinated axon

(c) would have its cell body only in the ventral (anterior) horn of the spinal cord

(d) might itself receive an input directly from group Ia afferent fibres in the spinal cord

(e) would be stimulated by application of glycine to its cell body

A125 (a) **F** As in nerve, tetrodotoxin blocks membrane sodium channels in skeletal muscle   **17.14**

(b) **T** Thiocyanate ions probably act on the T-tubules, facilitating transfer of excitation to the sarcoplasmic reticulum. Consequently Ca^{2+} release occurs at a smaller than normal level of depolarization during the action potential   **17.5, 17.15**

(c) **F** Caffeine does inhibit phosphodiesterase and it does potentiate contraction, but the two effects are not related; the latter property is due to Ca^{2+} release from the sarcoplasmic reticulum   **17.15**

(d) **T** The effect may be due to inhibition of uptake of Ca^{2+} by the sarcoplasmic reticulum, hence causing a prolongation of the active state   **17.15**

(e) **T** β-adrenoceptor agonists have similar effects. In thyrotoxicosis the origin of the tremor is complex; there are probably central components, effects of thyroid hormones on muscle cyclic AMP and synergism with catecholamines   **17.16**

A126 (a) **F** Each motoneurone innervates from 5 to several hundred muscle fibres — this forms the motor unit   **17.17**

(b) **T** Although the size of motoneurones ranges from large (α) to small (γ), the axons are all fast-conducting, myelinated fibres   **17.17**

(c) **F** Large numbers of motoneurones have cell bodies in the motor nuclei of the cranial nerves   **17.17**

(d) **T** This forms the monosynaptic reflex arc; the Ia afferents conduct impulses from the annulospiral (primary) sensory endings of the muscle spindles in the muscle innervated by the motoneurone   **6.2**

(e) **F** Glycine acts on receptors on motoneurone cell bodies to inhibit firing; this effect is blocked by strychnine   **14.16**

Q127 Blood flow in skeletal muscle:

(a) is decreased during isometric exercise of the participating muscles
(b) is decreased on cessation of exercise
(c) is facilitated through the veins by phasic contraction and relaxation of the muscle
(d) may be inadequate during fatigue, giving rise to ischaemic pain
(e) is predominantly under autonomic nervous control during muscular exercise

Q128 Competitive neuromuscular blocking agents:

(a) may be antagonized by a local increase in the concentration of acetylcholine
(b) block potassium-induced depolarization of skeletal muscle
(c) are antagonized by suxamethonium
(d) suppress both amplitude and duration of tetanic contractions of skeletal muscle
(e) are antagonized by hypothermia

A127 (a) **T** Sustained contraction mechanically compresses the blood vessels thus reducing their perfusion — **17.19**

(b) **F** On cessation of exercise there is a vasodilatation mediated by local metabolites which causes a brisk *increase* in flow. This phenomenon is called reactive hyperaemia — **17.20**

(c) **T** The transient vascular compression produced by contraction moves blood through the veins; the direction of bulk shift is towards the heart because the valves prevent retrograde flow. This phenomenon is known as the muscle pump — **23.23**

(d) **T** The pain occurs because inadequate vascular perfusion fails to clear one or more substances (probably produced by the contracting fibres) which stimulate afferent pain nerve endings — **17.19**

(e) **F** Vasomotor tone in exercising muscle is maintained at a low level by local vasodilators such as lactate and adenosine. These and possibly other vasodilator substances are produced by the contracting cells. The arterioles of exercising muscle are unresponsive to autonomic vasoconstrictors such as noradrenaline — **17.20, 23.20, 23.23**

A128 (a) **T** This is why they are described as competitive antagonists — **17.33**

(b) **F** They block only depolarization due to stimulation of nicotinic receptors by agonists — **17.34**

(c) **T** Suxamethonium competes for neuromuscular nicotinic receptors thereby displacing competitive antagonists, and causing membrane depolarization. This effect may summate with the effect of acetylcholine (the dose is critical since suxamethonium can cause blockade itself) — **17.35**

(d) **T** Tetanus generated by high frequency nerve stimulation depends upon build-up of acetylcholine in the cleft, thus tetanic amplitude is reduced by competitive antagonists; the marked reduction in duration is unexplained but clearly demonstrable — **17.35**

(e) **T** Probably because with lowered body temperature the rate of repolarization of the motor end plate is slowed and hence the depolarizing action of acetylcholine is enhanced — **17.36**

Q129 D-Tubocurarine (curare):

   (a)   is a competitive neuromuscular blocker
   (b)   causes a blockade which is intensified by neostigmine
   (c)   does not affect transmission in autonomic ganglia
   (d)   causes paralysis preceded by fasciculations of skeletal muscle
   (e)   produces a block at the motor end plate that is antagonized by potassium chloride

Q130 Suxamethonium:

   (a)   is a non-competitive neuromuscular blocking drug
   (b)   is a substrate for pseudocholinesterase
   (c)   depolarizes the motor end plate
   (d)   is used to assist endotracheal intubation
   (e)   after a single clinical dose produces a short-lasting (less than 10 minutes) paralysis in man

Q131 Considering polysynaptic reflexes:

   (a)   central summation is said to occur when preceding subliminal stimuli facilitate the ability of subsequent stimuli to activate the motoneurone
   (b)   stimulation of two sensory fibres together which excite the same motoneurone, always results in a doubling of the muscle tension produced
   (c)   the motoneurone pool is the group of motoneurones which may be activated by one interneurone
   (d)   the neuronal arrangement whereby a sensory nerve excites one muscle and inhibits the antagonist muscle is known as recruitment
   (e)   a crossed extensor reflex involves interneurones which cross the cord and excite the motoneurones supplying the contralateral limb

A129 (a) **T** It competes with acetylcholine for occupancy of motor end plate nicotinic receptors   **17.33**

(b) **F** Neostigmine inhibits acetylcholinesterase at the motor end plate, thus making available more acetylcholine to compete with D-tubocurarine. Neostigmine is used clinically to reverse competitive blockade   **17.36**

(c) **F** Although D-tubocurarine is *selective* towards motor end plate nicotinic receptors, it is not specific and will block nicotinic receptors in autonomic ganglia, especially at larger doses   **17.38**

(d) **F** This is true of suxamethonium which initially depolarizes end plates; D-tubocurarine does not   **17.43**

(e) **T** Potassium ions tend to depolarize the end plate, thereby facilitating transmission, hence end plate potentials produced by acetylcholine may summate and elicit an action potential more readily   **17.35**

A130 (a) **T** It binds to nicotinic receptors at the motor end plate in a non-competitive (with respect to acetylcholine) manner   **17.41**

(b) **T** Plasma pseudocholinesterase breaks down suxamethonium and limits its duration of action   **17.46**

(c) **T** Suxamethonium is a partial agonist; it first depolarizes the end plate and then blocks the receptors preventing further depolarization by acetylcholine   **17.41**

(d) **T** The short duration of action renders suxamethonium useful in paralysing the laryngeal muscles which would be activated briefly, but dramatically, by the cough reflex during endotracheal intubation   **17.46**

(e) **T** It has a short duration of action largely because of hydrolysis in plasma (see (b))   **17.46**

A131 (a) **T** Under some conditions the stimulus applied to the afferent fibre is too weak to depolarize the motor neurone (subliminal) but subsequent stimulation of the same sensory fibres or different fibres with the same final path, summate to activate the motor neurone   **18.2**

(b) **F** Facilitation or occlusion may occur, in which case the tension produced is either greater (facilitation) or less (occlusion) than when each fibre is stimulated separately   **18.3**

(c) **T** Many motoneurones receive synaptic connections from one interneurone — this explains how facilitation and occlusion (see (b)) can occur   **18.3**

(d) **F** This arrangement is known as reciprocal innervation — the antagonist is said to undergo reciprocal inhibition   **18.1**

(e) **T** At the same time, other interneurones inhibit the motoneurones to the antagonist muscles of the limb   **18.2**

Q132 With reference to the diagram:

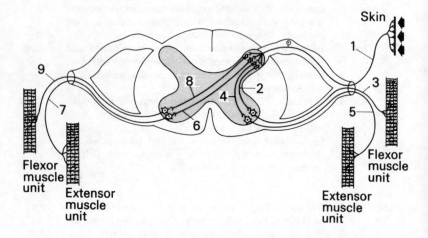

(a) stimulation of neurone 1 would tend to inhibit activity in neurone 3

(b) stimulation of neurone 1 would tend to inhibit activity in neurone 5

(c) stimulation of neurone 1 would tend to activate neurones 6 and 8

(d) stimulation of neurone 1 would tend to activate neurone 9

(e) stimulation of neurone 1 would tend to inhibit neurone 7

A132 (a) **F** Cutaneous afferent activation causes polysynaptic   **18.2**
                activation of the ipsilateral flexor neurones and forms
                the basis of the flexor reflex

(b) **T** Activation of the flexor muscle is associated with   **18.2**
          inhibition of the antagonist (extensor) muscle

(c) **T** Cutaneous afferent stimulation causes excitation of   **18.2**
          commissural interneurones

(d) **F** The crossed extensor reflex involves activation of the   **18.2**
          contralateral extensors by the same stimulus that
          causes ipsilateral flexor activation

(e) **F** Cutaneous afferent stimulation causes activation of   **18.2**
          contralateral extensors and inhibition of contralateral
          flexors

Q133 With reference to the diagram:

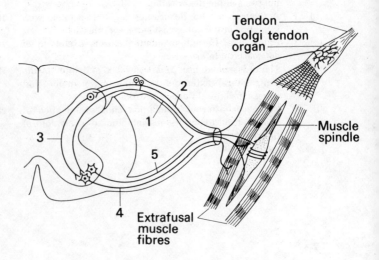

(a) activation of neurone 1 would induce monosynaptic reflex excitation of neurone 4

(b) activation of neurone 2 would cause excitation of neurone 4

(c) activation of neurone 5 would cause reflex activation of neurone 4

(d) activation of neurone 4 would tend to cause increased discharge in neurone 1

(e) activation of neurone 4 would tend to cause increased discharge in neurone 2

A133 (a) **T** This is the basis of the knee jerk reflex, for example. **18.6**
Stimulation of the annulospiral primary endings of the
muscle spindle (Ia afferents) elicits α-motoneurone
excitation

(b) **F** Neurone 2 is a Ib afferent associated with a Golgi-tendon **18.6**
organ; these fibres cause polysynaptic inhibition of α-
motoneurone activity

(c) **T** Stimulation of γ efferent fibres causes intrafusal muscle **18.6**
fibre contraction leading to activation of Ia afferents and
hence reflex excitation of α-motoneurones

(d) **F** Extrafusal muscle fibre contraction unloads the primary **18.6**
ending of the spindle and reduces its discharge

(e) **T** Contraction of extrafusal muscle fibres activates Golgi **18.6**
tendon organs

Q134 In man:

    (a)   efferent activity underlying voluntary movement is initiated in the motor cortex

    (b)   the number of neurones in the motor cortex representing the muscle groups for each part of the body is proportional to the size of the muscle group

    (c)   posture is maintained and adjusted mainly by the cerebellum

    (d)   diseases of the basal ganglia always result in hypo-kinetic states (infrequent spontaneous movement)

    (e)   damage to the cerebellum often results in intention tremor

Q135 The cerebellum:

    (a)   consists of an outer layer of white matter around the central grey matter

    (b)   receives afferent impulses from muscle spindles via second-order neurones whose axons run in the spinocerebellar tracts

    (c)   contains granule cells in the inner cortex which relay impulses from afferent (mossy) fibres to the Purkinje cells

    (d)   principally functions to achieve precise and smooth movement

    (e)   transmits efferent impulses along the axons of Purkinje cells to the lateral vestibular nuclei in the medulla

Q136 In normal man, the cerebellum:

    (a)   receives an afferent input from the cerebral cortex

    (b)   initiates activity in voluntary muscles

    (c)   receives an afferent input from the vestibular system

    (d)   provides an efferent output to the vestibular nuclei

    (e)   receives an ipsilateral input from muscle proprio-ceptors

A134 (a) **T** The principal motoneurones involved are called the   **18.8**
giant cells of Betz, the axons of which are myelinated
and up to 16 μm in diameter

(b) **F** The number of neurones is proportional to the   **18.9**
complexity of the movement, i.e. fingers, lips, vocal cords
are represented by large numbers compared to the
elbows, trunk and ankles

(c) **F** A system of neurones called the corticostrio-reticular   **18.8,**
system serves this function — it includes the corpus   **18.10**
striatum, substantia nigra, the red nucleus and the
reticular formation; there are also complex connections
with the motor cortex

(d) **F** The disorders arising from diseases of the basal ganglia   **18.11**
may be hypo- or hyper-kinetic

(e) **T** The cerebellum coordinates the body movements. When   **18.13**
diseased, an attempt to touch an object results in
overshoot and then overcompensation — this is known
as intention tremor

A135 (a) **F** The outer layer is grey matter and constitutes the cortex   **6.4**

(b) **T** These fibres synapse directly with the Purkinje cells in   **6.5,**
the outer (molecular) layer of the cortex   **18.4**

(c) **T** This is achieved either directly or through basket or   **6.5**
stellate cells

(d) **T** The cerebellum relates the actual position of the body to   **6.6,**
the intended position signalled by impulses from the   **18.12**
cerebral cortex; motion thus becomes precise and
smooth

(e) **T** Efferent impulses pass directly to these nuclei or via the   **6.6**
cerebellar nuclei to the reticular formation, red nuclei,
ventrolateral nucleus of the thalamus and thence to the
cerebral cortex

A136 (a) **T** This input relays in the pontine nuclei and projects to the   **6.7**
neocerebellum via the middle peduncles

(b) **F** The cerebellum coordinates movements initiated else-   **6.6**
where (including head and eye movements and the
activity of postural muscles)

(c) **T** This input projects to the archicerebellum via the   **6.7**
inferior peduncles

(d) **T** There is a direct and an indirect (via the fastigial   **6.7**
nucleus) output to the lateral vestibular nuclei (LVN)
from the archicerebellum and an indirect (via the
dentate nucleus) output to the LVN from the
neocerebellum

(e) **T** The spinocerebellar tracts convey afferent information   **6.15**
from proprioceptors to the cerebellum

Alimentary System

Q137 In normal man, saliva:

    (a)   secretion totals 2–3 l/day

    (b)   has a pH below 7 at low secretory rates

    (c)   contains α-amylase secreted by serous cells

    (d)   contains substances with characteristic antigenic structures

    (e)   contains an enzyme that initiates the digestion of protein

Q138 In normal man, saliva:

    (a)   is normally hypotonic with respect to plasma

    (b)   contains Na^+ at about the same concentration as in plasma

    (c)   contains K^+ at about the same concentration as in plasma

    (d)   contains HCO_3^- at about the same concentration as in plasma when secretory rate is maximal

    (e)   contains higher concentrations of electrolytes when the rate of secretion is high

Q139 In normal man, the salivary glands:

    (a)   respond to sympathetic stimulation by producing a secretion rich in α-amylase

    (b)   respond to parasympathetic stimulation by producing a secretion rich in mucins

    (c)   may be inhibited from secreting by tricyclic antidepressant drugs

    (d)   may be inhibited from secreting by neuroleptic phenothiazines

    (e)   may be inhibited from secreting by antihistamine drugs

A137 (a) **F** The total secretion is about 0.5–1.5 l (26% from parotid, 69% from submandibular, 5% from sublingual glands)   25.1

    (b) **T** Ordinary mixed saliva has a pH about 6.4, but as the rate of secretion rises the bicarbonate concentration increases and the pH rises   25.1

    (c) **T** The zymogen granules of the serous cells represent stored α-amylase   25.2

    (d) **T** Some of the mucopolysaccharides in saliva have the same antigenic structure as those conferring the blood groups   25.2

    (e) **F** Saliva contains α-amylase (which initiates the digestion of starches) and lysozyme (a bactericidal enzyme)   25.2

A138 (a) **T** The initial secretion is isotonic but becomes diluted due to reabsorption of electrolytes   25.2

    (b) **F** Na^+ concentration ranges from 5–90 mmol/l (versus about 140 mmol/l in plasma) due to reabsorption   25.2

    (c) **F** K^+ concentration is about 20 mmol/l (versus about 4.5 mmol/l in plasma) due to ductal secretion   25.2

    (d) **F** HCO_3^- concentration is about 60 mmol/l (versus about 24 mmol/l in plasma) under these conditions   25.2

    (e) **T** Presumably because the time for ductal reabsorption of secreted electrolytes is reduced   25.2

A139 (a) **F** Sympathetic stimulation produces viscid saliva rich in mucins   25.2

    (b) **F** Parasympathetic stimulation produces a copious saliva rich in α-amylase   25.2

    (c) **T** This effect has been attributed to a depressant action on the salivary centre in the medulla oblongata, or to generalized reduction in parasympathetic output (**15.17**)   25.2

    (d) **T** This is probably due to a peripheral anti-muscarinic action   25.2

    (e) **T** Such drugs frequently have atropine-like activity   25.2

Q140 In normal man, gastric motor activity is:

    (a)   abolished by bilateral gastric vagotomy
    (b)   inhibited by sympathetic nerve stimulation
    (c)   increased by cholecystokinin
    (d)   increased by secretin
    (e)   increased by alkalization of the duodenal contents

Q141 Vomiting may be:

    (a)   produced by stimulation of the vestibular system
    (b)   produced by stimulation of pain receptors associated with the genitalia
    (c)   inhibited by activation of the chemoreceptor trigger zone
    (d)   produced by apomorphine
    (e)   produced by phenothiazines

Q142 The parietal cells (oxyntic cells) of the gastric body and fundus:

    (a)   secrete a solution of hydrochloric acid which is nearly isosmotic with plasma
    (b)   show marked inhibition of secretion on treatment with carbonic anhydrase inhibitors
    (c)   secrete chloride ions passively into the gastric lumen
    (d)   when unstimulated, secrete acid at the rate of about 2 mmol/h in man
    (e)   when active cause a fall in the pH of gastric venous blood

A140 (a) **F** Vagotomy delays gastric emptying, but it does not abolish motor activity | 25.6

(b) **T** Sympathetic nerves inhibit activity of myenteric ganglion cells and some have a direct inhibitory effect on smooth muscle cells | 25.6

(c) **F** Fats entering the duodenum stimulate the release of cholecystokinin from the mucosa; this *inhibits* gastric motor activity and delays emptying | 25.20

(d) **F** Acidic chyme entering the duodenum stimulates secretin release from the proximal mucosa; this inhibits gastric motor activity | 25.20

(e) **T** This stimulates motilin release which enhances gastric motor activity | 25.20

A141 (a) **T** Activation of the inputs from semicircular canals, utricle and saccule is a potent stimulus for vomiting (motion sickness) | 25.7

(b) **T** Particularly with the epididymis (c.f. the term 'sickening pain') | 25.7

(c) **F** This region of the area postrema when stimulated causes vomiting and also has a tonic excitatory effect on the vomiting centre | 25.7

(d) **T** This drug when given intravenously is a powerful, centrally acting emetic (perhaps because of an agonist effect on central dopamine receptors) | 25.7

(e) **F** Many phenothiazines are anti-emetic although they tend to be less effective against labyrinthine than against other types of vomiting | 25.7

A142 (a) **T** The maximum hydrochloric acid concentration is about 150 mmol/l | 25.10

(b) **F** Although gastric acid secretion is reduced, it is not markedly inhibited because carbonic anhydrase levels are so high | 25.10

(c) **F** There are separate active transport mechanisms for hydrogen ions and chloride ions at the luminal surface | 25.10

(d) **T** When stimulated, the rate rises to about 25 mmol/h | 25.10

(e) **F** During acid secretion, HCO_3^- is added to gastric venous blood (in exchange for Cl^-) and hence pH rises | 25.10

Q143 In normal man, gastric juice:

(a) contains gastrin from the antral mucosa
(b) contains hydrochloric acid secreted by parietal cells
(c) totals 5–6 l/day
(d) has a pH in the range 5–6
(e) contains a proteolytic enzyme, pepsin

Q144 In normal man, gastric secretion:

(a) during the cephalic phase produces a juice rich in pepsin and acid
(b) in response to insulin-induced hypoglycaemia would be inhibited by ganglion-blocking drugs
(c) is stimulated by gastrin released mainly from the fundal mucosa
(d) is inhibited by histamine (H_2) receptor agonists
(e) is stimulated by muscarinic agonists

Q145 In normal man, gastric acid secretion is:

(a) stimulated by cholecystokinin released from the duodenal mucosa
(b) inhibited by secretin released from the duodenal mucosa
(c) stimulated by glucagon released from the α cells of the islets of Langerhans
(d) stimulated by histamine receptor (H_2) agonists
(e) stimulated by prostaglandin E_2

A143 (a) **F** Although this is the richest source of gastrin in the body, the hormone is secreted into the blood **25.10**

(b) **T** The secretion is similar to plasma with the exception that hydrogen ions replace sodium ions; the strength of the HCl is thus maximally about 150 mmol/l **25.10**

(c) **F** Normally the volume is 2–3 l/day **25.11**

(d) **F** Normally the range of pH is 1–2 **25.11**

(e) **T** This is derived from its precursor, pepsinogen, secreted by the peptic or chief cells of the gastric body and fundus **25.11**

A144 (a) **T** The efferent pathway is vagal to peptic and oxyntic cells and to gastrin-releasing cells; gastrin stimulates secretion of peptic and oxyntic cells **25.12**

(b) **T** A fall in blood glucose stimulates medullary preganglionic vagal efferent fibres to cause gastric secretion **25.12**

(c) **F** Gastrin is released mainly from the mucosa of the pyloric antrum **25.12**

(d) **F** Stimulation of H_2 receptors is probably the final common pathway in the excitation of parietal cells by all modes of activation **25.14, Fig. 25.7**

(e) **T** Muscarinic agonists stimulate parietal cell secretion (possibly via an H_2-receptor-mediated mechanism) and also elicit gastrin release which activates parietal cells **25.12**

A145 (a) **F** Cholecystokinin inhibits gastrin release and hence depresses gastric acid output **25.13**

(b) **T** Like cholecystokinin, secretin inhibits gastrin release and hence acid secretion **25.13**

(c) **F** Glucagon inhibits gastrin release and hence acid secretion **25.14**

(d) **T** H_2 receptor antagonists block gastric acid secretion and are becoming popular in the treatment of peptic ulcer **25.14**

(e) **F** Prostaglandin E_2 inhibits acid secretion in response to histamine or pentagastrin; inhibition of prostaglandin synthesis by aspirin may thus contribute to its ulcerogenic action **25.14**

Q146 The maximal gastric acid secretory response to penta-gastrin:

(a) is a reliable index of the presence of gastric ulceration

(b) is a useful test of the intactness of the vagal efferent supply to the stomach

(c) would be abnormal in an adult patient with pernicious anaemia

(d) is, on average, greater in men than in women

(e) would be inhibited in the presence of an antihistamine such as mepyramine

Q147 Peptic ulceration:

(a) may be produced by anti-inflammatory analgesics such as salicylates

(b) may be effectively treated with glucocorticoids

(c) may be effectively treated with histamine (H_2) antagonists such as cimetidine

(d) may be healed by treatment with sodium bicarbonate

(e) leading to persistent vomiting, may produce hypokalaemia

Q148 The duodenal contents may include:

(a) a trypsin-like enzyme

(b) high levels of cholecystokinin when the pH is high

(c) high levels of secretin when the pH is below 7

(d) α-amylase

(e) enzymes that hydrolyse nucleic acids

A146 (a) **F**   Gastric acid secretion may be below normal in many patients with gastric ulcer (possibly because acid is reabsorbed across the damaged mucosa)   **25.17**

(b) **F**   Pentagastrin is a synthetic analogue of gastrin; it stimulates parietal cells via a mechanism not involving neural elements   **25.12**

(c) **T**   Gastric mucosal atrophy leads to loss of parietal cells and hence absence of acid secretion and intrinsic factor (the latter is necessary for the absorption of vitamin B_{12} which is involved in erythropoiesis)   **21.37**

(d) **T**   The maximal response is an estimate of parietal cell mass; in men it averages 23, and in women 16 mmol/h   **25.16**

(e) **F**   Antihistamines are H_1 antagonists and do not affect acid secretion   **25.16**

A147 (a) **T**   Possibly because inhibition of prostaglandin synthesis disinhibits gastric acid secretion   **25.17**

(b) **F**   Glucocorticoids have an ulcerogenic action   **25.17**

(c) **T**   Substantial healing of peptic ulcers is effected with cimetidine, presumably due to inhibition of gastric acid secretion   **25.18**

(d) **F**   Antacids have little effect on healing — they only relieve symptoms associated with peptic ulceration   **25.18**

(e) **T**   Gastric juice is high in potassium ions that are normally reabsorbed; with vomiting, potassium is lost from the body   **28.25**

A148 (a) **T**   Brunner's glands secrete a precursor that is activated by HCl and which then hydrolyses peptide links made by lysine   **25.20**

(b) **F**   The presence of fats or amino acids stimulates the release of cholecystokinin from the duodenal mucosa into the bloodstream — not into the lumen   **25.20**

(c) **F**   In response to acid chyme, secretin is released into the bloodstream — not into the lumen   **25.20**

(d) **T**   This enzyme is secreted by the acinar cells of the pancreas and reaches the duodenum through the pancreatic duct   **25.22**

(e) **T**   Ribonuclease and deoxyribonuclease which hydrolyse RNA and DNA respectively are secreted by the pancreas and drain into the duodenum   **25.22**

Q149 In normal man, cholecystokinin:

    (a)   is released from the mucosa of the distal duodenum in response to a fall in luminal concentrations of amino acids

    (b)   stimulates the release of bile into the duodenum

    (c)   release is inhibited by the presence of trypsin in the duodenum

    (d)   stimulates the release of trypsinogen from the pancreas

    (e)   stimulates the release of gastrin

Q150 In normal man, secretin:

    (a)   is released by the mucosa of the proximal duodenum in response to a rise in luminal pH

    (b)   stimulates pancreatic secretion containing high bicarbonate concentrations

    (c)   inhibits the secretion of bicarbonate into bile

    (d)   stimulates the release of pepsinogen from the gastric mucosa

    (e)   decreases gastrin release

Q151 In normal man, excitation of vagal efferent fibres:

    (a)   may cause an enzyme-rich secretion from pancreatic acinar cells

    (b)   inhibits insulin release from pancreatic β cells

    (c)   inhibits contraction of the gall bladder

    (d)   stimulates gastrin release

    (e)   inhibits secretion of gastric acid

A149 (a) **F** Cholecystokinin release is stimulated by amino acids in the duodenum   25.20

(b) **T** Cholecystokinin stimulates gall-bladder contraction and relaxation of the sphincter of Oddi   25.20

(c) **T** Cholecystokinin stimulates enzyme-rich pancreatic secretion which, in turn, inhibits cholecystokinin secretion (negative feedback)   25.20

(d) **T** Cholecystokinin in the blood has potent stimulatory effects on secretion of trypsinogen by pancreatic acini   25.20

(e) **F** In man, cholecystokinin inhibits gastrin release, although the terminal octapeptide has gastrin-like activity   25.20

A150 (a) **F** Secretin release is stimulated by the entry of acid chyme into the duodenum   25.20

(b) **T** Secretin stimulates pancreatic acinar cells and epithelial cells of the ducts — the latter are the source of the secreted HCO_3^- 25.20

(c) **F** Secretin stimulates bile secretion and this is associated with increased HCO_3^- secretion   25.20

(d) **T** Pepsinogen gives rise to pepsin (by autocatalysis in acid media), a proteolytic enzyme   25.21

(e) **T** And hence reduces acid output; this would tend to reduce conversion of pepsinogen to pepsin (an example of negative feedback control — see (d))   25.21

A151 (a) **T** Vagal efferent fibres provide an excitatory innervation for pancreatic acinar cells   25.21

(b) **F** The vagal innervation of pancreatic β cells is excitatory   19.49

(c) **F** The vagal innervation of the gall-bladder is excitatory   25.21

(d) **T** The vagal innervation of gastrin-secreting cells is excitatory   25.15

(e) **F** Acetylcholine directly stimulates the parietal cells; in addition, it promotes the release of gastrin from the mucosal cells of the antrum which then stimulates gastric acid secretion   25.12

Q152 In normal man, pancreatic juice:

(a) totals about 2 l/day

(b) contains high concentrations of bicarbonate

(c) entering the duodenum stimulates the release of secretin

(d) contains inactive precursors of proteolytic enzymes

(e) is the sole source of lipase

Q153 In the gastrointestinal tract:

(a) water may be reabsorbed throughout its length

(b) sodium is reabsorbed actively by a process sensitive to aldosterone

(c) proteins are absorbed in the form of dipeptides

(d) the products of fat digestion are absorbed mainly in the ileum

(e) fat malabsorption may be produced by neomycin

Q154 Peristaltic movements of the small intestine:

(a) are initiated by activity in the central nervous system

(b) may be elicited in an isolated segment of intestine by raising the intraluminal pressure

(c) may be stimulated by α-adrenoceptor agonists

(d) may be stimulated by nicotinic receptor antagonists

(e) would be inhibited by muscarinic receptor antagonists

Q155 In the large intestine:

(a) sugars and amino acids may be absorbed

(b) stimulation of extrinsic parasympathetic nerves causes excitation which is inhibited by nicotinic receptor antagonists

(c) pain due to colic may be treated with morphine alone

(d) up to 50% of the contents may be bacterial in origin

(e) the gas present is largely that swallowed with the food

144   *Alimentary System*

A152	(a)	F	The secretory rate is normally about 1 l/day	25.22
	(b)	T	The bicarbonate is probably secreted by the epithelial cells of the ducts	25.22
	(c)	F	Secretin release is stimulated by a fall in duodenal pH — pancreatic juice has a pH about 8	25.20
	(d)	T	For example, trypsinogen is initially activated by enzymatic hydrolysis (involving enterokinase) and the activation is continued by trypsin	25.22
	(e)	F	A lipase is also secreted in the duodenum and jejunum	25.25

A153	(a)	T	Water moves in association with reabsorbed sodium, so that gut contents tend to be isotonic with plasma	25.26
	(b)	T	Epithelial sodium transport in the gut, as in sweat glands and the kidney, is sensitive to aldosterone	25.26
	(c)	F	Proteins are completely hydrolysed to L-amino acids which are actively absorbed	25.26
	(d)	F	Absorption only occurs in the small intestine, but mainly in the duodenum and jejunum	25.26
	(e)	T	Neomycin inhibits intestinal lipase and thus reduces fat digestion	25.26

A154	(a)	F	Peristaltic activity is initiated by local events, but may be modulated by central nervous activity	25.27
	(b)	T	This stimulates sensory nerve endings, and elicits the co-ordinated activity that is dependent on the intrinsic nerve plexuses	25.27
	(c)	F	Alpha-adrenoceptor agonists act on cell bodies in the myenteric plexus and cause inhibition	25.28
	(d)	F	Excitatory transmission through the intrinsic plexuses is blocked by nicotinic receptor antagonists	25.28
	(e)	T	Reflex excitation of the smooth muscle depends on neuronally released acetylcholine acting on muscarinic receptors	25.28

A155	(a)	T	Although they are not normally present they can be absorbed, thus nutrition can be achieved by introducing such substances into the rectum	25.29
	(b)	T	The extrinsic nerves to the colon are, in part excitatory, and are preganglionic	25.31
	(c)	F	Morphine causes an increase in intracolonic pressure which may exacerbate the problem; morphine plus an atropine-like agent relieves the pain and lowers intra-colonic pressure	25.31
	(d)	T	Apart from indigestible components of the food, cell debris and mucin, the remainder is bacterial in origin	25.32
	(e)	F	The majority of gas present is generated by bacterial fermentation	25.32

Q156 In normal man, constipation:

(a) is defined as a frequency of defaecation of less than once every three days

(b) may be produced by the narcotic analgesic morphine

(c) may be produced by the neuroleptic phenothiazines

(d) may be alleviated by sympathomimetic agents

(e) may be produced by the anticholinesterase neostigmine

Q157 Laxatives and purgatives:

(a) include the bulk laxative cellulose

(b) include the lubricant laxative, castor oil

(c) include the irritant purgative, phenolphthalein

(d) include the saline purgative, magnesium sulphate

(e) should be used routinely to prevent absorption of toxins from the colon

Q158 In normal man, resting, in the overnight fasted state:

(a) the liver receives about 30% of the cardiac output

(b) the hepatic arterial blood flow is about 1.2 l/min

(c) the portal venous blood flow is about 1.2 l/min

(d) the maintenance of hepatic function is largely dependent on portal venous blood

(e) portal venous pressure is less than hepatic arterial pressure, due to the low resistance of hepatic sinusoids

A156 (a) **F** It depends on diet and habit; a change in frequency may be of clinical significance   25.32

(b) **T** It increases the tone of the anal sphincter and decreases propulsive movements; the central actions of the drug may reduce awareness of the need to defaecate   16.4

(c) **T** These drugs have atropine-like and ganglion-blocking activities; both would contribute to a constipating action   25.33

(d) **F** Stimulation of α or β-adrenoceptors relaxes intestinal smooth muscle; the former action also inhibits ganglion cell activity in the myenteric plexus   25.33

(e) **F** Anticholinesterases enhance the action of cholinergic excitatory nerves and thus tend to produce diarrhoea   25.37

A157 (a) **T** Cellulose is undigested and hence increases faecal weight, decreases intestinal transit time and increases the frequency of defaecation   25.33

(b) **F** Castor oil acts as an irritant purgative; although in itself it is non irritant, it is hydrolysed by intestinal lipase to liberate ricinoleic acid which produces intense stimulation of peristalsis   25.35

(c) **T** Phenolphthalein acts as an irritant purgative by stimulating peristalsis in the colon (possibly by acting on sensory endings); in addition it inhibits glucose absorption in the small intestine (thus possibly having a 'bulk' effect)   25.36

(d) **T** Such substances are poorly absorbed in the gut and so exert an osmotic effect drawing water into the gut; they may cause dehydration   25.34

(e) **F** There is no evidence that this normally occurs   25.32

A158 (a) **T** Resting cardiac output is about 5.0 l/min, hepatic blood flow is about 1.5 l/min   26.1

(b) **F** The hepatic artery carries about 20% of the total flow, i.e. about 0.3 l/min   26.1

(c) **T** The portal vein delivers about 80% of the total blood flow, i.e. about 1.2 l/min   26.1

(d) **F** In spite of supplying the majority of blood perfusing the liver, portal venous blood is less important than hepatic arterial blood for the nutrition of the liver   26.1

(e) **F** Portal venous pressure is low due to the vascular resistance of the beds through which the blood has drained before reaching the portal vein   26.1

Q159 In the normal liver:

(a) glucose is synthesized from amino acids and fatty acids only

(b) utilization of blood glucose is stimulated by insulin

(c) glycogenolysis may provide glucose as a substrate for exercising muscle

(d) plasma albumin is synthesized at a rate of 10–12 g per day

(e) all the fat-soluble vitamins are stored

Q160 In normal man, bile:

(a) when first secreted by the hepatocytes is hypotonic to plasma

(b) contains pigments that are mostly synthesized in the liver

(c) contains bile salts that are necessary for the digestion of fats

(d) flow may be impaired by neuroleptic phenothiazines

(e) flow is increased by fats in the duodenum

Q161 In man jaundice may be produced by:

(a) antimalarial drugs, such as chloroquine

(b) neuroleptic phenothiazines, such as chlorpromazine

(c) anticoagulant drugs, such as phenindione

(d) the diuretic drug frusemide

(e) the antibiotic novobiocin

A159 (a) **F** The synthesis of glucose from lactate plays an important role in maintaining blood glucose during exercise, for example   26.3

(b) **T** Liver cells take up glucose by a process that is insensitive to insulin, but subsequent metabolism is insulin dependent   19.45

(c) **T** Hepatic glycogenolysis produces glucose that passes into the blood; this may then undergo glycolysis in the exercising muscle (the lactate produced may act as a precursor for hepatic glucose synthesis)   2.19

(d) **T** Hence hepatic disorders give rise to reduction in colloid osmotic pressure and a tendency to oedema   26.4

(e) **T** Vitamins A, D, E and K; the water-soluble vitamins cyanocobalamin and folic acid are also stored in the liver   26.4

A160 (a) **F** Hepatic bile is roughly isotonic, is secreted at the rate of 250–1200 ml/day and is temporarily held in the gall-bladder where it is concentrated up to tenfold by reabsorption of water and electrolytes. However, this does not increase the tonicity of the bile because the salts, pigments, lecithin and cholesterol form micelles which have low osmotic activity   26.4

(b) **F** They are catabolic products of haem which is largely synthesized in erythroblasts   26.4

(c) **T** The bile salts are secreted into the duodenum where they emulsify fats and activate pancreatic lipase   26.8

(d) **T** For example, chlorpromazine; simple precipitation of bile glycoproteins with chlorpromazine may contribute to the plugging of biliary canaliculi   26.33

(e) **T** This stimulates cholecystokinin release which elicits gall-bladder contraction   25.20

A161 (a) **T** Chloroquine may cause haemolytic anaemia (**21.46**); the destruction of erythrocytes produces bilirubin at a rate in excess of the liver's ability to glucuronidate it and levels in plasma and tissues rise   26.7

(b) **T** Chlorpromazine reacts with some component (glycoproteins) of bile and precipitates in the canaliculi, obstructing outflow and thus gives rise to elevated systemic levels of biliary constituents   26.7

(c) **T** Oral anticoagulants act on liver cells as vitamin K antagonists; phenindione may cause damage to hepatocytes, leading to jaundice   26.33

(d) **T** Bilirubin binds to plasma albumin; frusemide competes for the binding sites and displaces bilirubin giving rise to elevated tissue levels   26.7

(e) **T** Novobiocin inhibits bilirubin glucuronyl transferase and hence causes elevated bilirubin levels, particularly in babies   26.8

Q162 In normal man, the bile acids:

(a)   deoxycholic acid and lithocholic acid are formed in the liver by the oxidation of cholesterol

(b)   in the form of their salts, are largely reabsorbed in the lower ileum

(c)   are secreted at a greater rate in the presence of secretin

(d)   in the form of their salts, hold cholesterol in solution

(e)   in the form of their salts, stimulate bile secretion

A162 (a) **F** Cholic acid and chenodeoxycholic acid are formed in the   **26.9**
liver; lithocholic and deoxycholic acid are formed in the
intestine by a bacterial enzyme acting on the primary
bile acids

(b) **T** About 90% (20–30 g/day) of the bile salts secreted are   **26.8**
taken up in the lower ileum, enter the portal venous
blood and are secreted again into bile; the liver is
capable of synthesizing new bile salts at the rate of
3–5 g/day only

(c) **F** Secretin stimulates hepatic secretion of water and   **25.20**
electrolytes without any increase in the secretion of bile
salts or pigments (c.f. its effects on the pancreas)

(d) **T** These highly surface-active molecules form macromole-   **26.80**
cular aggregates with lecithin (micelles) which dissolve
cholesterol

(e) **T** Bile salts act directly on liver parenchymal cells to stimu-   **26.10**
late bile secretion

Kidney

Q163 In the kidneys:

(a) all glomeruli lie in the cortex
(b) proximal tubular cells have a brush border on their luminal surface
(c) about 45% of the nephrons lie in the cortex and have short loops
(d) about 15% of the nephrons have long loops
(e) afferent arterioles are longer and narrower than most arterioles

Q164 In the kidneys:

(a) the efferent arterioles generally have a smaller diameter than the afferent arterioles
(b) the majority of renin-secreting cells lie in the walls of the efferent arterioles
(c) the blood flow normally amounts to about 10% of the cardiac output
(d) of a normal man, the plasma flow is about 700 ml/min
(e) efferent arterioles of juxtamedullary nephrons give rise to vasa recta

Q165 The glomerular filter:

(a) consists of capillary endothelial cells joined by tight junctions
(b) is freely permeable to water
(c) is freely permeable to protein
(d) is impermeable to haemoglobin
(e) actively transports electrolytes

A163 (a) **T** Most of the glomeruli are located in the superficial part of the cortex; only about 15% are located near the junction of the cortex and medulla   **27.2**

    (b) **T** This suggests they are adapted for absorption (the enzyme carbonic anhydrase is found in association with the brush border (**27.8**))   **27.1**

    (c) **F** About 85% of the nephrons are cortical   **27.2**

    (d) **T** These juxtamedullary nephrons have loops that extend deep into the medulla   **27.2**

    (e) **F** Afferent arterioles are shorter and wider than is usual; as a result glomerular capillary hydrostatic pressure is higher than capillary hydrostatic pressure elsewhere   **27.3**

A164 (a) **T** The higher efferent resistance helps maintain glomerular capillary hydrostatic pressure   **27.3**

    (b) **F** The granular cells are mainly in the walls of the afferent arterioles (hence intrarenally generated angiotensin II may act on efferent vessels)   **27.3**

    (c) **F** Under resting conditions, renal blood flow is about 25% of the cardiac output   **27.3**

    (d) **T** Renal blood flow is approximately 25% of the cardiac output (5 l/min), i.e. 1250 ml/min. Thus with an average haematocrit of 45%, this gives a renal plasma flow of [(55 × 1250)/100] ml/min, i.e. 700 ml/min   **27.3**

    (e) **T** These vessels act as countercurrent exchangers and help to maintain the medullary concentration gradient   **27.3**

A165 (a) **F** The glomerular capillary endothelium is fenestrated   **27.3**

    (b) **T** The composite barrier does not exclude water molecules   **27.3**

    (c) **F** Very little plasma protein normally gets into the filtrate   **27.3**

    (d) **F** Haemoglobin passes the filter, although normally it is not able to since it is enclosed in erythrocytes   **27.3**

    (e) **F** The glomerular filter acts as a semi-permeable membrane   **27.4**

Q166 The sympathetic innervation of the kidney:

(a) supplies afferent arterioles

(b) supplies efferent arterioles

(c) supplies granular cells in the walls of the afferent arterioles

(d) when stimulated electrically, is likely to cause an increase in urine formation

(e) when reflexively activated always causes a decrease in glomerular filtration rate

Q167 The glomerular filtration rate:

(a) would be increased if glomerular capillary hydrostatic pressure fell

(b) would be increased if the hydrostatic pressure in Bowman's capsule rose

(c) would be increased if plasma colloid osmotic pressure were reduced

(d) would be increased if efferent arterioles constricted

(e) would be increased if afferent arterioles constricted

Q168 In a normal man over 24 hours:

(a) about 180 l of glomerular filtrate are formed

(b) about 5 l of urine are excreted

(c) about 0.5–1% of the sodium filtered is excreted

(d) about 0.5–1% of the potassium filtered is excreted

(e) about 30–40 mg of plasma albumin are excreted

A166 (a) **T**   Activation causes afferent constriction and a fall in glomerular filtration rate   **27.3**

(b) **T**   Activation causes efferent constriction and a rise in glomerular filtration rate   **27.3**

(c) **T**   Activation may cause renin release independent of vascular events   **27.3**

(d) **F**   Electrical stimulation tends to cause a fall in renal blood flow and hence urine formation   **27.3**

(e) **F**   When reflex efferent constriction is more marked than afferent constriction, glomerular filtration rate rises   **27.3**

A167 (a) **F**   The glomerular capillary hydrostatic pressure provides a driving force for filtrate formation   **27.4**

(b) **F**   Capsular pressure acts to reduce filtration   **27.4**

(c) **T**   Colloid osmotic pressure opposes filtration   **27.4**

(d) **T**   This would act to raise glomerular capillary hydrostatic pressure   **27.4**

(e) **F**   This would act to lower glomerular capillary hydrostatic pressure and thus hinder filtration   **27.4**

A168 (a) **T**   Glomerular filtration rate is about 125 ml/min, thus daily glomerular filtrate is $(125 \times 60 \times 24)$ ml   **27.5**

(b) **F**   Normally about 1.5 l of urine are passed daily   **27.5**

(c) **T**   In normal man on a normal sodium intake, sodium balance is well maintained, with output equalling intake, i.e. 100–250 mmol/day   **27.5**

(d) **F**   Plasma potassium (4.5 mmol/l) is much lower than sodium (140 mmol/l) thus the filtered load of potassium (810 mmol/day) is much smaller than that of sodium (25 mol/day); in balance, about 80 mmol of potassium are excreted per day, i.e. about 10% of the filtered load   **27.5**

(e) **T**   The glomerular filter is more or less impermeable to albumin, so only very small amounts get through (about 36 g are filtered per day); much of the protein filtered is reabsorbed by pinocytosis   **27.5**

Q169 In the proximal convoluted tubule:

    (a)   about 20% of the filtrate is reabsorbed

    (b)   water movements are primarily influenced by antidiuretic hormone

    (c)   most of the filtered potassium is reabsorbed

    (d)   filtered protein is reabsorbed

    (e)   all filtered glucose is reabsorbed

Q170 In the proximal convoluted tubule:

    (a)   glucose reabsorption is impaired by inhibitors of ATP synthesis

    (b)   glucose reabsorption is unimpaired in the presence of other sugars

    (c)   amino acid transport depends on genetically determined enzymes

    (d)   at birth the amino acid reabsorption processes are not fully functional

    (e)   sodium is passively reabsorbed

Q171 In the proximal convoluted tubule:

    (a)   the sodium concentration in the lumen is about half that in the interstitial fluid

    (b)   luminal and peritubular surfaces are freely permeable to potassium

    (c)   about 10% of the filtered chloride is reabsorbed

    (d)   about 70% of the filtered phosphate is reabsorbed

    (e)   urea is passively reabsorbed

A169	(a)	F	About 80% of the filtrate is reabsorbed — largely due to active sodium reabsorption	27.5
	(b)	F	Antidiuretic hormone only affects the water permeability of the distal convoluted tubule and collecting duct; water reabsorption in the proximal tubule follows the active transport of sodium	27.5
	(c)	T	Potassium is actively transported independently of sodium	27.7
	(d)	T	Although little protein is filtered, that which is undergoes reabsorption by pinocytosis, mainly in the proximal tubule	27.7
	(e)	F	This is true if the filtered load does not exceed the transport maximum for glucose	27.5

A170	(a)	T	There is an active transport of glucose that is sodium dependent (as in the intestine)	27.5
	(b)	F	Other sugars compete for the 'carrier' mechanism	27.5
	(c)	T	Certain rare hereditary diseases are associated with an inability to reabsorb some amino acids	27.5
	(d)	T	The delayed development of these mechanisms gives rise to loss of amino acids in neonatal urine	27.6
	(e)	F	Sodium is actively reabsorbed by a process probably associated with the lateral peritubular borders of the cells	27.7

A171	(a)	F	Sodium reabsorption gives rise to passive water movements, so the luminal and interstitial sodium concentrations are the same	27.7
	(b)	T	Potassium is actively pumped into the cells at both surfaces and diffuses out	27.7
	(c)	F	About 80% of the chloride is reabsorbed; reabsorption is largely passive, mainly in association with sodium	27.7
	(d)	T	There is an inverse relation between glucose and phosphate reabsorption; this is possibly due to a common energy source or to a mutual sodium dependency	27.7
	(e)	T	The reabsorption of sodium and water concentrates the urea in the luminal fluid and it moves down this concentration gradient	27.11

Q172 In the proximal tubule:

(a) parathyroid hormone (PTH) impairs the reabsorption of phosphate

(b) parathyroid hormone (PTH) impairs the reabsorption of calcium

(c) vitamin D metabolites decrease the reabsorption of calcium

(d) the net reabsorption of sodium is influenced by the colloid osmotic pressure in the peritubular capillaries

(e) about 140 l of filtrate are reabsorbed daily

Q173 In the proximal tubule:

(a) the luminal surface is freely permeable to bicarbonate

(b) the reabsorption of bicarbonate is enhanced by carbonic anhydrase

(c) bicarbonate reabsorption acts to correct systemic acidosis

(d) there is no net addition of hydrogen ion to the tubular fluid

(e) bicarbonate reabsorption would be decreased by a drug that inhibited sodium reabsorption

Q174 In the loop of Henle:

(a) the descending limb is freely permeable to water

(b) the thin ascending limb is freely permeable to water

(c) an active chloride pump is localized in the thick ascending limb

(d) the fluid at the end of the thick ascending limb is always hypotonic

(e) the fluid at the tip is normally hypertonic

A172 (a) **T** This effect involves a parallel inhibition of sodium and bicarbonate reabsorption, and thus may be due to a primary effect on sodium reabsorption **27.7**

(b) **F** PTH enhances calcium reabsorption by an action which involves stimulation of adenylate cyclase **19.68**

(c) **F** Vitamin D metabolites stimulate the synthesis of a calcium carrier protein, thereby playing a permissive role in the action of PTH **19.68**

(d) **T** Increased peritubular colloid osmotic pressure facilitates capillary reabsorption and reduces backflux into the proximal tubule **27.4**

(e) **T** 80% of the filtrate (total about 180 l/day) is absorbed proximally **27.5**

A173 (a) **F** The luminal membrane is impermeable to filtered HCO_3^-; the net reabsorption of HCO_3^- depends on the intracellular generation of HCO_3^- **27.7**

(b) **T** Carbonic anhydrase facilitates the production of luminal carbon dioxide; this carbon dioxide diffuses into the cells and is involved in the generation of HCO_3^- **27.8**

(c) **F** The HCO_3^- reabsorbed is that which was filtered and thus cannot offset acidosis; HCO_3^- generated distally may contribute to the correction of acidosis **27.8**

(d) **T** The H^+ secreted is 'recycled' in the reabsorption of HCO_3^-, so does not contribute to H^+ excretion in the definitive urine **27.8**

(e) **T** HCO_3^- reabsorption is passive and associated with sodium reabsorption **27.8**

A174 (a) **T** Osmotic extraction of water from the fluid in the descending limb makes the fluid progressively more hypertonic as it reaches the tip of the loop **27.8**

(b) **F** This portion is relatively impermeable to water; sodium chloride reabsorption at this site and in the thick ascending limb (unaccompanied by water) generates the hypotonic fluid that passes into the distal convoluted tubule **27.8**

(c) **T** This pump adds chloride (and, passively, sodium) to the interstitium making it hypertonic; it is this hypertonic solution which causes osmotic extraction of water from the fluid in the descending limb **27.8**

(d) **T** This is due to the reabsorption of chloride (and sodium) unaccompanied by water **27.8**

(e) **T** The countercurrent multiplier mechanism generates increasing concentration in tubular and interstitial fluids deep in the medulla (up to 1200 mosmol/kg in man) **27.8**

Q175 In the distal convoluted tubule:

(a)   increased sodium delivery facilitates potassium secretion

(b)   aldosterone acts to enhance sodium reabsorption

(c)   aldosterone acts to enhance potassium reabsorption

(d)   antidiuretic hormone (ADH) acts to increase water permeability

(e)   antidiuretic hormone (ADH) acts to increase urea permeability

Q176 In the distal convoluted tubule:

(a)   there is an active secretion of hydrogen ions

(b)   the secretion of hydrogen ions is enhanced by buffering with phosphate in the luminal fluid

(c)   the secretion of hydrogen ions is reduced when ammonia levels in the luminal fluid are increased

(d)   about 50% of the filtered bicarbonate is reabsorbed

(e)   the majority of the bicarbonate reabsorbed is generated intracellularly

Q177 Antidiuretic hormone (ADH):

(a)   increases the water permeability of the distal convoluted tubule and the collecting duct

(b)   is released in response to a rise in extracellular volume

(c)   is released in response to a fall in plasma osmolality

(d)   has a pressor action which is exerted at lower plasma levels than its antidiuretic action

(e)   is released from nerve terminals in the posterior pituitary gland

A175 (a) **T** Probably due to an increased sodium diffusion potential at the luminal surface facilitating the passive secretion of potassium   27.9

(b) **T** Probably by increasing the efficiency or number of sodium pumps   27.9

(c) **F** Aldosterone enhances potassium excretion by a mechanism separate from that of its effects on sodium reabsorption — possibly by increasing luminal permeability to potassium   27.9

(d) **T** In the presence of ADH water moves out of the tubules, thus reducing the volume of urine   27.10

(e) **F** ADH only affects the urea permeability of the medullary portion of the collecting duct   27.11

A176 (a) **T** These are generated from carbonic acid intracellularly, thus this mechanism eliminates H^+ and adds HCO_3^- to the body   27.10

(b) **T** The reaction is $H_2PO_4^- \rightleftharpoons HPO_4^{2-} + H^+$ and the pKa is 6.8; when the pH of urine is 7.4, $HPO_4^{2-}:H_2PO_4^-$ is 4:1 but when the pH falls to 6.8 $HPO_4^{2-}:H_2PO_4^-$ is 1:1; thus the amount of H^+ buffered increases as the pH falls   27.10, 28.21

(c) **F** Generation of NH_3 from glutamine facilitates H^+ secretion by buffering $(NH_3 + H^+ \rightleftharpoons NH_4^+)$ 27.10

(d) **F** Very little filtered HCO_3^- remains (the majority is reabsorbed in the proximal tubule)   27.10

(e) **T** The H^+ actively secreted derives from H_2CO_3 generated intracellularly leaving HCO_3^- that fluxes into the blood $(H_2O + CO_2 \rightleftharpoons H_2CO_3 \rightleftharpoons H^+ + HCO_3^-)$ 27.10

A177 (a) **T** ADH stimulates adenylate cyclase and processes involving microtubules, although the actual mechanism of the change in water permeability is unclear   27.10, 27.11

(b) **F** A reduction in blood volume unloads cardiopulmonary and arterial baroreceptors and this increases ADH release   27.10

(c) **F** A fall in plasma osmolality inhibits ADH release possibly acting via hypothalamic osmoreceptors   19.13

(d) **F** Although ADH is a potent vasocontrictor its antidiuretic effects are normally expressed at lower plasma levels than those that have overt cardiovascular effects   19.14

(e) **T** The cells of origin are largely in the paraventricular nucleus   19.14

Q178 In the kidney:

    (a)   the urea present is formed largely in the liver

    (b)   urea excretion is influenced by urine flow

    (c)   uric acid is actively reabsorbed in the proximal convoluted tubule

    (d)   the final concentration of the urine is achieved in the collecting duct

    (e)   the vasa recta actively maintain the medullary concentration gradient

Q179 Renal plasma flow (RPF)

    (a)   varies directly with systemic arterial pressure

    (b)   is mainly directed through the cortex

    (c)   in haemorrhage, tends to decrease more than glomerular filtration rate (GFR)

    (d)   is the rate-limiting step in para-aminohippuric acid (PAH) secretion at low (< 0.2 mmol/l) plasma levels of PAH

    (e)   divided by glomerular filtration rate is termed the filtration fraction

Q180 During an investigation of renal function in a normal patient, the following measurements were made: ante-cubital venous plasma PAH concentration = 0.1 mmol/l; rate of urine production = 120 ml/h; urine PAH concentration = 32 mmol/l; inulin clearance = 125 ml/min; antecubital venous plasma protein concentration = 70 g/l; packed cell volume = 45%. From these values it follows:

    (a)   PAH excretion rate was 3.84 mmol/h

    (b)   the effective renal plasma flow (ERPF) was 840 ml/min

    (c)   the effective renal blood flow (ERBF) was 1163 ml/min

    (d)   the filtration fraction was 0.40

    (e)   the plasma protein concentration in the efferent arterioles would have been about 87 g/l

A178	(a)	**T**	It derives from the ammonia generated from the deamination of amino acids	**27.11**
	(b)	**T**	Slower tubular flow rates permit longer time for passive reabsorption and vice versa	**27.11**
	(c)	**T**	Some is also secreted, but the bulk is reabsorbed	**27.11**
	(d)	**T**	Osmotic water extraction in the presence of ADH produces a concentrated urine and vice versa	**27.11**
	(e)	**F**	The vasa recta act as passive countercurrent exchangers	**27.11**
A179	(a)	**F**	Autoregulatory mechanisms operate to maintain blood flow approximately constant in man over a range of perfusion pressures from 70–200 mmHg	**23.20**
	(b)	**T**	The majority of nephrons and the associated vasculature lie in the cortex	**27.2**
	(c)	**T**	More pronounced efferent than afferent constriction tends to maintain GFR	**27.3**
	(d)	**T**	These levels at normal renal plasma flows (about 700 ml/min) present the transport mechanism with 0.14 mmol/min; the transport maximum for PAH is about 0.4 mmol/min	**27.13**
	(e)	**F**	The filtration fraction indicates the proportion of plasma filtered and is equal to GFR/RPF	**27.14**
A180	(a)	**T**	The excretion rate is equal to the urine concentration (32 mmol/l) multiplied by the urine flow rate (0.12 l/h)	**27.13**
	(b)	**F**	The ERPF = PAH clearance, i.e. (urine PAH concentration × urine volume)/plasma PAH concentration = 640 ml/min	**27.13**
	(c)	**T**	The ERBF = ERPF/(1-packed cell volume), i.e. 1163 ml/min	**27.13**
	(d)	**F**	The filtration fraction = GFR/ERPF = 125/640 = 0.20	**27.13**
	(e)	**T**	Protein is not filtered so the original mass of protein (70 g/l) remains in the blood that passes into the efferent arterioles, thus there would be 70 g in 800 ml (given a filtration fraction of 0.20), i.e. 87.5 g/l	**27.14**

Q181 During an investigation of renal function a patient was infused with a solution of glucose and inulin and the following observations were made:

Plasma inulin concentration	= 0.1 mmol/l
Plasma glucose concentration	= 20 mmol/l
Urine inulin concentration	= 2.6 mmol/l
Urine glucose concentration	= 120 mmol/l
Urine flow rate	= 300 ml/h

From these figures it follows that:

(a) the inulin clearance was 75 ml/min
(b) the glucose clearance was 30 ml/min
(c) the amount of glucose filtered was 2.6 mmol/min
(d) the amount of glucose excreted was 6 mmol/min
(e) the transport maximum for glucose reabsorption was 4 mmol/min

Q182 In a hypothetical experiment the following observations with regard to renal function were made:

PAH clearance	= 280 ml/min
Osmolal clearance	= 8 ml/min
Albumin clearance	= 2 ml/min
Glucose clearance	= 50 ml/min
'x' clearance	= 13 ml/min

(a) the PAH clearance indicates that renal plasma flow was abnormally low
(b) low osmolal clearance indicates that the urine would have been hypotonic
(c) the albumin clearance indicates renal abnormality
(d) the glucose clearance indicates abnormal renal handling of glucose
(e) the clearance of 'x' indicates that it must have been reabsorbed

A181 (a) **F**   Inulin clearance = (urine inulin concentration × urine   **27.13**
volume)/plasma inulin concentration = (2.6 × 5)/0.1 =
130 ml/min

(b) **T**   Glucose clearance = (120 × 5)/20 = 30 ml/min   **27.13**

(c) **T**   Glucose filtered = GFR × plasma glucose concentration   **27.14**
= 0.13 × 20 = 2.6 mmol/min

(d) **F**   Glucose excreted = urine glucose concentration × urine   **27.14**
volume
= 120 × 0.005 = 0.6 mmol/min

(e) **F**   Transport maximum for glucose = quantity filtered −   **27.14**
quantity excreted, i.e. 2.6 − 0.6 = 2 mmol/min

A182 (a) **F**   At high plasma concentrations the T_m for PAH is   **27.14**
exceeded and the clearance falls towards that for inulin
even in the presence of normal renal function

(b) **F**   The tonicity of the urine depends on the ratio of osmoles   **27.15**
to water molecules and cannot be deduced from this
figure

(c) **T**   Normally very little albumin is filtered and clearance is   **27.6**
about 0.02 ml/min; the value given indicates a 'leaky'
filter

(d) **F**   At high plasma glucose levels the T_m for glucose is   **27.14**
exceeded and glucose is excreted, giving a positive
clearance

(e) **F**   Clearance values below that of inulin may be taken as an   **27.13**
indication of reabsorption only if the substance is freely
filtered − 'x' may not be

Q183 Oedema may occur in response to:

(a) a chronic reduction in cardiac output
(b) a reduction in hepatic protein synthesis
(c) hyposecretion of aldosterone
(d) increased glomerular capillary permeability to protein
(e) increased dietary protein intake

Q184 The carbonic anhydrase inhibitor acetazolamide:

(a) depresses the reabsorption of bicarbonate in the proximal tubule
(b) increases the reabsorption of sodium in the proximal convoluted tubule
(c) increases the secretion of potassium in the distal convoluted tubule
(d) gives rise to a metabolic alkalosis
(e) has a diuretic action which is most marked with repeated dosing

Q185 The thiazide diuretic hydrochlorthiazide:

(a) acts by inhibiting reabsorption in the thick ascending limb of the loop of Henle
(b) causes a reduction in plasma aldosterone levels
(c) reduces potassium loss in the urine
(d) may be used in the treatment of arterial hypertension
(e) inhibits active sodium reabsorption by the renal tubule

168 *Kidney*

A183 (a) **T** In congestive heart failure the reduction in cardiac 27.27
output is 'sensed' as a decrease in effective blood volume
and mechanisms come into play to increase blood
volume; fluid retention and the increased capillary
filtration pressure tends to shift water and electrolytes
into the tissue spaces

(b) **T** Plasma proteins are synthesized in the liver; a reduction 27.27
in this process gives rise to a fall in plasma colloid
osmotic pressure and increased formation of tissue fluid

(c) **F** Hyposecretion of aldosterone would be likely to lead to 27.27
volume depletion; hypersecretion of aldosterone pro-
duces sodium retention leading to extracellular volume
expansion

(d) **T** This leads to a reduction in plasma colloid osmotic 27.27
pressure and loss of fluid from the vascular compartment into the interstitium

(e) **F** *Decreased* protein intake leads to reduced hepatic 27.27
protein synthesis and hence oedema formation

A184 (a) **T** The luminal membrane is impermeable to HCO_3^- so net 27.30
HCO_3^- reabsorption depends on $H^+ + HCO_3^- \rightleftharpoons H_2CO_3 \rightleftharpoons CO_2 + H_2O$; the latter reaction is catalysed by carbonic
anhydrase

(b) **F** The non-reabsorbed bicarbonate holds sodium in the 27.30
tubule and reduces its net reabsorption

(c) **T** The increased presentation of sodium to distal sites 27.30
facilitates potassium secretion

(d) **F** Loss of bicarbonate and the failure to generate HCO_3^- 27.30
distally gives rise to a metabolic acidosis

(e) **F** The metabolic acidosis it produces limits its action 27.30
because there is a reduced mass of filtered bicarbonate
and sufficient H^+ available to effect its reabsorption
without the action of carbonic anhydrase

A185 (a) **F** Thiazides do not affect the corticomedullary concentra- 27.33
tion gradient, so it is unlikely that they interfere with this
process

(b) **F** The hyponatraemia due to sodium loss and the 27.33
accompanying hypovolaemia cause hyperaldosteronism

(c) **F** It causes potassium loss, largely as a result of increased 27.33
presentation of sodium to the distal tubular reabsorptive
site, facilitating potassium secretion

(d) **T** The antihypertensive action is probably due to volume 27.33
contraction and peripheral vasodilatation — possibly
due to phosphodiesterase inhibition

(e) **T** The site of action is most likely the 'diluting segment' of 27.32
the distal tubule, i.e. proximal to the aldosterone
sensitive site

Q186   The diuretic drug frusemide:

    (a)   causes a marked inhibition of bicarbonate reabsorption

    (b)   inhibits active chloride reabsorption in the thick ascending limb of the loop of Henle

    (c)   interferes with the urine concentrating mechanism

    (d)   is a more potent diuretic than hydrochlorthiazide

    (e)   increases potassium loss in the urine

Q187   A drug that acts as a competitive antagonist of aldosterone:

    (a)   is likely to cause metabolic alkalosis

    (b)   may cause hyperkalaemia

    (c)   is likely to have an enhanced diuretic effect in a patient on a high sodium intake

    (d)   will have a more potent diuretic effect than frusemide

    (e)   would be the first choice in treating primary (essential) hypertension

Q188   The osmotic diuretic mannitol:

    (a)   inhibits active sodium reabsorption in the proximal tubule

    (b)   reduces bicarbonate reabsorption in the proximal tubule

    (c)   increases proximal tubular reabsorption of urea

    (d)   impairs the ability to excrete a concentrated urine

    (e)   increases distal tubular potassium secretion

A186 (a) **F** Frusemide acts at a site distal to the proximal tubule (which is where the majority of filtered HCO_3^- is reabsorbed)   27.35

(b) **T** This is its main site of action   27.35

(c) **T** Inhibition of Cl^- reabsorption dissipates the medullary concentration gradient so the osmotic extraction of water from collecting duct fluid is reduced   27.35

(d) **T** Interference with the medullary concentration gradient and inhibition of Cl^- transport can produce urine flow rates of as much as 10 l/day; hydrochlorthiazide is less potent since it does not affect the medullary concentration gradient   27.35

(e) **T** The increased presentation of sodium to the distal tubule facilitates potassium secretion   27.35

A187 (a) **F** It is likely to interfere with the distal tubular secretion of H^+ and hence cause metabolic acidosis   27.35

(b) **T** It will inhibit distal tubular potassium secretion and hence may produce hyperkalaemia   27.35

(c) **F** Under these conditions aldosterone levels would be low and a competitive antagonist would have a reduced effect   27.35

(d) **F** The mechanism interfered with handles less sodium chloride than that inhibited by frusemide; also it does not influence the urine-concentrating mechanism   27.35

(e) **F** Such a drug would be an unlikely choice in the treatment of hypertension of any origin — they are only mild diuretics and they are expensive   27.35

A188 (a) **F** It inhibits passive water reabsorption and thereby increases the backflux of sodium so reducing net sodium reabsorption   27.36

(b) **T** The reduction in proximal tubular reabsorption of sodium inhibits the passive reabsorption of bicarbonate   27.36

(c) **F** The reabsorption of urea is passive and dependent on the reabsorption of sodium; it would, therefore, be decreased   27.36

(d) **T** The reduced water reabsorption leads to high tubular flow rates and an impairment of the action of ADH   27.36

(e) **T** Increased presentation of sodium to the distal tubule and the high distal tubular flow rate facilitate potassium secretion   27.36

Q189 Renin:

   (a)   is released from the granules of juxtaglomerular cells of the afferent arteriole
   (b)   levels in blood increase in response to a fall in plasma sodium concentration
   (c)   levels in blood decrease when renal perfusion is reduced
   (d)   release is enhanced by angiotensin II
   (e)   release is inhibited by ADH

Q190 Considering the renin–angiotensin–aldosterone system:

   (a)   angiotensinogen (renin substrate) is a protein
   (b)   renin acts on angiotensinogen to produce aldosterone
   (c)   about 90% of angiotensin I is converted to angiotensin II in the lungs
   (d)   angiotensin II is a potent vasodilator
   (e)   angiotensin II stimulates aldosterone release from the adrenal medulla

Q191 Considering the renin–angiotensin–aldosterone system:

   (a)   aldosterone release is inhibited by a fall in plasma potassium
   (b)   angiotensin II may cause increased fluid intake
   (c)   angiotensin II facilitates noradrenaline release from noradrenergic nerves
   (d)   angiotensin II facilitates catecholamine release from the adrenal medulla
   (e)   the responses to angiotensin II are terminated by its uptake into lung tissue

A189 (a) **T** These are modified smooth muscle cells   **12.28**

     (b) **T** Possibly as a response to the reduced presentation of sodium to the macula densa   **12.28**

     (c) **F** When renal perfusion falls, renin release increases; this is possibly due to decreased stretch of the afferent arteriole   **12.28**

     (d) **F** Renin release is inhibited by angiotensin II (thus forming a negative feedback loop)   **12.28**

     (e) **T** There is some evidence that this may be a direct effect of ADH on the juxtaglomerular cells   **12.28**

A190 (a) **T** It is an α_2-globulin synthesized (largely) in the liver   **12.28**

     (b) **F** Renin converts angiotensinogen to the decapeptide angiotensin I   **12.28**

     (c) **T** The converting enzyme responsible for this process is found mostly in the lungs   **12.28**

     (d) **F** Angiotensin II is a very potent vasoconstrictor (particularly in the skin, kidney and intestines)   **12.28**

     (e) **F** Aldosterone is released from the zona glomerulosa of the adrenal cortex   **12.28**

A191 (a) **T** Potassium directly affects aldosterone release from the zona glomerulosa; a rise in plasma potassium increases aldosterone levels in blood, thus promoting renal potassium excretion   **12.29**

     (b) **T** Angiotensin II stimulates the thirst centre and causes drinking   **6.28**

     (c) **T** It is possible that in volume-depleted states this mechanism together with a direct vasoconstrictor action, serves to maintain blood pressure   **12.29**

     (d) **T** This action occurs at sub-pressor plasma levels of angiotensin II   **12.29**

     (e) **F** The most important factor for terminating the response to angiotensin II is uptake into tissues but the only organ which does not seem to be involved in this process is the lung   **12.29**

Q192 In a normal adult in normal conditions during 24 hours:

    (a)   about 0.1 l of water is lost in expired air
    (b)   between 0.1–8.0 l of water may be lost in sweat
    (c)   about 2.0 l of water are lost in faeces
    (d)   about 4.0 l of water are lost in urine
    (e)   the minimum total water loss is about 1.8 l

Q193 In a normal subject, water intake below that necessary to compensate for losses would give rise to:

    (a)   an increased plasma sodium concentration
    (b)   excretion of reduced amounts of sodium in the urine
    (c)   reduced levels of antidiuretic hormone in blood
    (d)   reduced angiotensin II levels in blood
    (e)   excretion of a hypotonic urine

Q194 In a normal subject water intake in excess of loss:

    (a)   would cause an increase in extracellular fluid (ECF) volume only
    (b)   would cause a more marked diuresis than the same excess intake in the form of isotonic saline
    (c)   would cause a marked increase in packed cell volume (PCV)
    (d)   would lead to a decrease in urinary osmolality
    (e)   would lead to an increase in mean corpuscular volume

A192 (a) **F** Normally about 0.4 l of water is lost this way; the value 28.6
may be much higher if ventilation rate is increased

(b) **T** This depends on the ambient temperature; in high 28.6
temperatures, thermoregulatory sweating can reach
enormous rates

(c) **F** Gut fluid is extensively reabsorbed in the colon so that 28.6
about 0.2 l of water is normally lost in faeces

(d) **F** On a normal diet (with a normal fluid intake) the 28.6
obligatory water loss in the urine is about 1.0 l

(e) **T** Taking minimal values for all losses; the working range 28.6
for clinical purposes is taken to be 1.8–2.2 l/day under
basal conditions

A193 (a) **T** If sodium-free water is lost, this must concentrate the 28.7
plasma sodium

(b) **T** The hypovolaemia resulting from dehydration would 28.7
activate sodium-conserving mechanisms

(c) **F** The hypovolaemia and the hyperosmolality would both 28.7
stimulate ADH release

(d) **F** The hypovolaemia stimulates renin release giving rise to 28.7
increased formation of angiotensin II

(e) **F** Sodium retention would give rise to low sodium in the 28.7
urine, but ADH-mediated water reabsorption relative to
other solutes would give rise to a hypertonic urine

A194 (a) **F** The water would distribute throughout the body since 28.8
addition to the ECF would dilute this compartment
relative to the intracellular fluid volume (ICF) and water
would move into cells

(b) **T** Isotonic saline would cause no change in ECF or ICF 28.8
osmolality; water causes ECF (and ICF) dilution and this,
together with the ECF expansion (albeit smaller than
with saline which stays in the ECF) is a more potent
stimulus for inhibition of ADH release

(c) **F** Although erythrocytes swell under these conditions the 28.8
volume of blood occupied by the cells stays about the
same since the plasma volume is also increased

(d) **T** The ECF dilution and expansion both act to inhibit ADH 28.8
release and hence lead to increased water excretion

(e) **T** Water would enter erythrocytes to achieve osmotic 28.8
equilibrium

Q195 A female whose total body water was 35 kg (20 kg intracellular, 15 kg extracellular) ingested (and retained) 2 kg of solute-free water. Assuming the initial osmolality of her body fluids was 280 mosmol/kg:

    (a)   the initial total body solute was 9800 mosmol
    (b)   the initial extracellular solute was 4200 mosmol
    (c)   the new osmolality of body fluids would have been 250 mosmol/kg
    (d)   the new mass of ECF would have been 16.5 kg
    (e)   the new mass of ICF would have been 20.5 kg

Q196 In a normal subject, sodium depletion unaccompanied by a corresponding loss of water would lead to:

    (a)   plasma hyperosmolality
    (b)   an increase in ICF volume
    (c)   a decrease in ECF volume
    (d)   a more marked reduction in plasma than in interstitial volume
    (e)   a decrease in packed cell volume

Q197 In a patient in whom sodium intake exceeded sodium output:

    (a)   there would be an increase in ECF volume
    (b)   there would be a decrease in ICF volume
    (c)   there would be an increase in plasma colloid osmotic pressure
    (d)   there would be an increase in the packed cell volume (PCV)
    (e)   aldosterone levels would be low, normally

A195 (a) **T** 35 kg × 280 mosmol/kg = 9800 mosmol   **28.8**
    (b) **T** 15 kg × 280 mosmol/kg = 4200 mosmol   **28.8**
    (c) **F** Calculated from new total body water (35 + 2) and the   **28.8**
total body solute which would not have changed (9800
mosmol), then the new osmolality = 9800/37, i.e. 265
mosmol/kg
    (d) **F** Calculated from extracellular solute (4200) and the new   **28.8**
osmolality (265) the new mass of extracellular fluid
would have been 15.84 kg
    (e) **F** Calculated from the difference between the new total   **28.8**
body water (37 kg) and the new extracellular water
(15.84 kg) it would have been 21.16 kg; from intracellular solute (5600) and the new osmolality (265) it
would have been 21.13 kg

A196 (a) **F** Sodium loss would tend to cause hypoosmolality, but this   **28.9**
would inhibit ADH release and tend to normalize
osmolality
    (b) **T** Persistent sodium loss evokes water retention (to   **28.9**
maintain ECF volume) and the dilution of ECF causes a
fluid shift into cells (but see (a))
    (c) **T** Due to water flux into cells as a result of the relative   **28.9**
hyperosmolality of the ICF
    (d) **F** The fall in plasma volume would lead to a rise in colloid   **28.9**
osmotic pressure and a shift of fluid from the interstitium
to the vascular compartment, so the interstitial volume
would be reduced more than the vascular volume
    (e) **F** Increased ICF together with reduced plasma volume   **28.9**
would cause marked increases in packed cell volume

A197 (a) **T** The increased osmolality would cause fluid to shift from   **28.10**
cells. ADH secretion would be increased to maintain
osmolality and fluid would be retained
    (b) **T** This is due to the osmotic shift of water since the excess   **28.10**
sodium does not get into cells (being excluded by the
sodium pump)
    (c) **F** Plasma protein concentration would be diluted by the   **28.10**
addition of protein-free fluid to the ECF
    (d) **F** Reduction in intracellular water and increase in plasma   **28.10**
volume would reduce PCV
    (e) **T** High ECF volume and sodium load should inhibit renin   **28.10**
release and ultimately aldosterone release — unless
hyperaldosteronism was the problem

Q198 The following values were found in an arterial blood sample from a patient: P_{CO_2} = 22 mmHg; pH = 7.35; HCO_3^- = 12 mmol/l. From these values it follows that:

(a) the primary disturbance is likely to have been respiratory

(b) there would have been increased excretion of NH_4^+ in the urine

(c) plasma potassium levels are likely to have been high

(d) the majority of the phosphate excreted would have been in the form of HPO_4^{2-}

(e) the low P_{CO_2} would have acted to inhibit peripheral chemoreceptor drive to ventilation

Q199 The following values were found in an arterial blood sample from a patient: P_{CO_2} = 20 mmHg; pH = 7.5; HCO_3^- = 15 mmol/l. From these values it follows that:

(a) the primary disturbance is likely to have been metabolic

(b) there would have been increased sodium excretion in the urine

(c) there would have been decreased potassium excretion in the urine

(d) there would have been decreased NH_4^+ excretion in the urine

(e) the patient is likely to have had raised aldosterone levels

A198 (a) **F** Hyperventilation would cause a rise in pH but here pH is lower than normal   28.2

(b) **T** In severe sustained metabolic acidosis as much as 500 mmol/day NH_4^+ may be excreted   28.2

(c) **T** Prolonged acidosis of either respiratory or metabolic origin may cause hyperkalaemia due to decreased potassium ion excretion and displacement of intracellular potassium ion by H^+ 28.2

(d) **F** In an acid urine, virtually all phosphate excreted is in the $H_2PO_4^-$ form, the reaction $HPO_4^{2-} + H^+ \rightleftharpoons H_2PO_4^-$ being an important buffer system   28.21

(e) **T** The ventilatory response would be due to central chemoreceptor drive (H^+) balanced by inhibition of peripheral drive (due to hypocapnia)   28.21

A199 (a) **F** The decreased HCO_3^- is consistent with a metabolic acidosis but here the patient is alkalotic, so the low HCO_3^- is due to renal compensation for respiratory alkalosis   28.2

(b) **T** Reduced reabsorption of HCO_3^- would reduce sodium ion reabsorption   28.25

(c) **F** Reduced H^+ secretion and increased sodium presentation to the distal tubule would facilitate potassium secretion   28.25

(d) **T** Increased HCO_3^- excretion raises urine pH and inhibits the NH_4^+ production mechanism ($NH_3 + H^+ \rightleftharpoons NH_4^+$) and less H^+ is secreted   28.25

(e) **T** Sodium ion loss (with HCO_3^-) leading to hyponatraemia and hypovolaemia would activate the renin-angiotensin–aldosterone system   28.25

Q200 The following values were found in an arterial blood sample from a patient: P_{CO_2} = 80 mmHg; pH = 7.35; HCO_3^- = 45 mmol/l. From these values it follows that:

(a) the primary disturbance is likely to have been respiratory

(b) the disturbance is likely to have existed for some days

(c) there would have been large amounts of HCO_3^- in the urine

(d) urine volume would have been elevated

(e) plasma potassium concentration would have been decreased

Q201 The following values were found in an arterial blood sample from a patient: P_{CO_2} = 42 mmHg; pH = 7.6; HCO_3^- = 40 mmol/l. From these values it follows that:

(a) the primary disturbance is likely to have been metabolic

(b) the patient is likely to have been volume depleted

(c) the disorder is likely to have arisen as a result of increased renal HCO_3^- reabsorption

(d) the patient is likely to have been hyperkalaemic

(e) the patient is likely to have had reduced plasma ionized calcium ion levels

A200 (a) **T** If the primary disturbance had been metabolic alkalosis, the respiratory compensation would have been moderate and pH would have been above 7.4 28.20

(b) **T** The elevation of plasma HCO_3^- depends on the renal generation of HCO_3^- and is influenced by the induction of the ammonium mechanism which takes some days 28.20

(c) **F** Renal HCO_3^- reabsorption would be maximal and little HCO_3^- would be excreted 28.20

(d) **F** Elevated HCO_3^- reabsorption would tend to cause sodium ion retention and hence decreased urine volume 28.20

(e) **F** Elevated distal tubular H^+ secretion would interfere with potassium ion secretion and increased H^+ in the body might lead to displacement of intracellular potassium ion — these effects would tend to cause hyperkalaemia 28.20

A201 (a) **T** HCO_3^- is raised and the patient is alkalotic; the raised P_{CO_2} as a primary disturbance would produce an acidosis 28.20

(b) **T** The increased HCO_3^- excretion would be accompanied by sodium causing sodium and water loss 28.25

(c) **F** Normally, almost all filtered HCO_3^- is reabsorbed, so the renal addition of HCO_3^- to the body depends on HCO_3^- generation associated with H^+ secretion; the only ways the present disorder could come about is by ingestion of HCO_3^-, loss of gastric H^+ (by vomiting for example), rapid correction of chronic respiratory acidosis, or with diuretic therapy (the induced sodium and water loss resulting in elevation of HCO_3^- due to reduction in its volume of distribution) 28.20

(d) **F** H^+ secretion would be reduced and potassium secretion increased; furthermore potassium would enter cells due to reduced intracellular levels of H^+ and increased HCO_3^- 28.26

(e) **T** Due to the rise in plasma pH, calcium ionization would be reduced 28.25, 28.30

Q202 Considering potassium in the body:

(a) plasma levels influence aldosterone secretion
(b) plasma levels may be influenced by insulin
(c) elevated levels may produce metabolic alkalosis
(d) plasma levels provide a good index of potassium balance
(e) hypokalaemia may lead to oedema

Q203 Considering calcium in the body:

(a) hypocalcaemia produces hypoexcitability of the neuromuscular system
(b) hypercalcaemia may lead to renal damage
(c) hypercalcaemia may occur in hyperparathyroidism
(d) the amount filtered by the kidneys depends on plasma pH
(e) diuretics such as frusemide may be used to treat hypercalcaemia

A202	(a)	T	Elevated plasma potassium levels stimulate aldosterone secretion and thereby increase renal potassium excretion	19.35
	(b)	T	In the presence of insulin (and glucose) cellular uptake of potassium is increased	28.26
	(c)	F	Elevated plasma potassium concentration suppresses H^+ secretion, which would produce metabolic acidosis	28.26
	(d)	F	Loss of potassium from plasma causes efflux of potassium from cells (down the concentration gradient); thus plasma potassium levels may be 'normal' in the face of a deficit in total body potassium content	28.27
	(e)	T	Hypokalaemia may reduce cardiac inotropy and thereby reduce cardiac output; the subsequent events are similar to those seen with congestive heart failure	28.27

A203	(a)	F	Loss of the stabilizing action of calcium on nerve and muscle membranes causes hyperexcitability	28.30
	(b)	T	The increased filtered load of calcium may give rise to calcium precipitation in tubules, etc.	28.31
	(c)	T	PTH releases calcium from bone and promotes its tubular reabsorption	28.31
	(d)	T	Binding of calcium to plasma proteins depends on pH; when bound it is not freely filtered	28.30
	(e)	T	Loop diuretics increase the renal elimination of calcium; this is because in the proximal tubule and medullary ascending limb (but not the cortical ascending limb or the distal tubule), active Ca^{2+} reabsorption is linked to Na^+ transport	28.30

Reproductive System

Q204 In the human testis:

    (a)   spermatogenesis takes place in the seminiferous tubules

    (b)   spermatozoa arise directly from germ cells (spermatogonia)

    (c)   Sertoli cells regulate spermatogenesis

    (d)   follicle stimulating hormone (FSH) stimulates spermatogenesis by increasing the protein content of Sertoli cells

    (e)   spermatogenesis only occurs at normal deep body temperature

Q205 In the human male:

    (a)   spermatogenesis is inhibited if testicular temperature falls below deep body temperature

    (b)   the cells of Sertoli in the seminiferous tubules can synthesize androgens

    (c)   spermatozoa are derived from spermatogonia by mitosis

    (d)   spermatogenesis is stimulated by FSH

    (e)   vitamin A is essential for spermatogenesis

A204 (a) **T** Spermatogenic cells line the seminiferous tubules; those **20.2**
on the basement membrane ultimately give rise to sper-
matozoa

(b) **F** Spermatogonia divide into A cells and B cells. The B cells **20.2**
then differentiate into primary spermatocytes which, in
turn, form secondary spermatocytes, spermatids and
eventually spermatozoa

(c) **T** The intracellular lipid content of Sertoli cells is deter- **20.2**
mined by the rate of spermatogenesis; when this content
rises above a certain level, the Sertoli cells somehow
inhibit spermatogenesis

(d) **F** FSH reduces the intracellular lipid concentration of **20.2**
Sertoli cells thereby removing the inhibitory influence on
spermatogenesis

(e) **F** Spermatogenesis occurs at temperatures 1–3 °C below **20.2**
that of the abdominal cavity

A205 (a) **F** The testes are normally 1–3 °C below abdominal cavity **20.2**
temperature and the scrotum is well adapted to maintain
this lower temperature since spermatogenesis is
inhibited at higher temperatures

(b) **T** Although the cells of Sertoli are mainly concerned with **20.2**
the regulation of spermatogenesis, they have the
capacity to synthesize sex steroids; the interstitial cells
of Leydig, which occur in groups in the connective tissue
between the seminiferous tubules, usually synthesize
androgens

(c) **F** Spermatogonia divide mitotically to produce type A and **20.2**
type B cells; the latter differentiate into primary spermatocytes that divide meiotically, producing secondary
spermatocytes. These divide mitotically to produce spermatids that mature into spermatozoa

(d) **T** FSH from the adenohypophysis acts on the cells of **20.2**
Sertoli to reduce intracellular lipid levels; this, in some
way, disinhibits division of spermatogonia

(e) **T** Deficiency of vitamin A results in atrophy of the ger- **20.3**
minal cells. The conversion of retinol (the form in which
vitamin A is ingested) to the active aldehyde form
(retinal) is dependent on a dehydrogenase in testicular
tissue

Q206 In the human male:

(a) the production of testosterone is stimulated by FSH

(b) the release of interstitial cell stimulating hormone (ICSH) begins at puberty

(c) testosterone inhibits release of interstitial cell stimulating hormone (ICSH) from the pituitary

(d) the adrenal synthesis of androgens is stimulated by adrenocorticotrophin (ACTH)

(e) hypogonadism is most effectively treated with anabolic agents such as nandrolone

Q207 Testosterone:

(a) is mainly produced in the cells of Sertoli

(b) is produced only in the testis

(c) production is stimulated by luteinizing hormone (LH)

(d) halts linear growth

(e) is produced from androstenedione partly in the liver

Q208 In the adult female:

(a) Fallopian tubes convey ova from the ovaries to the uterus

(b) the segment of the Fallopian tube closest to the ovary is called the ampulla

(c) the uterus and connective tissue capsules of the ovaries are connected by broad ligaments

(d) the middle layer of the uterus is muscular

(e) the structure of the inner layer of the uterus varies during the menstrual cycle

A206 (a) **F**   The cells of Sertoli synthesize testosterone under the   **20.3**
influence of ICSH; FSH stimulates spermatogenesis

     (b) **T**   ICSH from the adenohypophysis at puberty stimulates   **20.3**
the production of androgens which cause maturation of
the genitalia and the development of secondary sexual
characteristics

     (c) **T**   Testosterone and other androgens inhibit ICSH release   **20.4**
from the adenohypophysis — probably by suppressing
the formation of its hypothalamic releasing factor

     (d) **T**   Androstenedione and dehydroepiandrosterone are pro-   **20.4**
duced in the adrenal cortex, and their conversion to
testosterone also occurs in the liver. Adrenal synthesis is
enhanced by ACTH from the adenohypophysis

     (e) **F**   Hypogonadism indicates an androgen deficiency which   **20.6**
should be made good by androgen administration (e.g.
fluoxymesterone). Anabolic agents are used to treat
conditions in which protein wasting has occurred; these
drugs have relatively little androgenic action

A207 (a) **F**   The cells of Leydig (interstitial cells) are mainly responsi-   **20.3**
ble for the production of steroid hormones

     (b) **F**   The ovary and adrenal cortex produce small amounts of   **20.4**
testosterone

     (c) **T**   LH (identical to ICSH) is produced in the anterior pitui-   **20.3**
tary and stimulates the production of testosterone

     (d) **T**   Testosterone causes bone maturation and fusion of the   **20.4**
epiphyses

     (e) **T**   Androstenedione and dihydroepiandrostenedione   **20.3**
(which are formed in the adrenal cortex, ovary and
testis) are converted to testosterone within the glands
that produce them, and in the liver

A208 (a) **T**   The ovum is picked up by the infundibular fimbriae and   **20.9**
conveyed to the ampulla where fertilization takes place
(when it does); muscular activity then conveys the ovum
to the uterus

     (b) **F**   The Fallopian tube is divided into 4 segments; infundi-   **20.9**
bulum (closest to ovary), ampulla, isthmus and uterine
(interstitial) portions

     (c) **F**   The broad ligaments connect the outer surface of the   **20.9**
uterus to the body wall; ovarian ligaments connect the
uterus to the ovarian capsules

     (d) **T**   This is called the myometrium; in the cervical region the   **20.9**
bundles of muscle fibres are predominantly circularly
disposed and form a sphincter

     (e) **T**   The endometrium undergoes cyclical changes of   **20.9,**
destruction and regeneration under the influence of   **20.21**
ovarian hormones

Q209 In the human ovary:

    (a)   ovarian follicles are formed during fetal life

    (b)   each ovarian follicle contains several primordial ova

    (c)   the zona granulosa is formed from proliferating follicle cells

    (d)   FSH causes the mature Graafian follicle to rupture

    (e)   the ovum is released into the Fallopian tube

Q210 In the human female:

    (a)   the production of ovarian follicles is stimulated by FSH at puberty

    (b)   ovulation occurs when rupture of the follicle is stimulated by LH

    (c)   during early pregnancy, the corpus luteum produces large amounts of oestradiol

    (d)   progesterone enhances renal sodium reabsorption

    (e)   oral ingestion of small amounts of progesterone leads to infertility

Q211 Progesterone:

    (a)   is produced by the developing ovarian follicle

    (b)   transforms the endometrium into a secretory endothelium

    (c)   enhances the contractile response of the myometrium to oxytocin

    (d)   is produced by the placenta throughout pregnancy

    (e)   is metabolized mainly in the liver

A209 (a) **T** Of the 500 000 that are formed, about 500 mature in adult life   **20.10, 20.38**

(b) **F** Each follicle contains only one ovum surrounded by follicular cells   **20.10**

(c) **T** This surrounds the ovum and lines the antrum   **20.10**

(d) **F** The process, known as ovulation, is stimulated by LH; FSH promotes follicle development   **20.10**

(e) **F** The ovum is released into the abdominal cavity and is swept into the Fallopian tube by the ciliary activity of cells of the fimbriae at the mouth of the tube   **20.10**

A210 (a) **F** The ovarian follicles are formed during fetal life; at puberty FSH stimulates the proliferation of follicular cells and the conversion of ovarian into Graafian follicles   **20.10**

(b) **T** LH is probably identical with ICSH; it is secreted by the adenohypophysis. It induces ovulation by stimulating rupture of the mature follicle and also promotes the conversion of the remaining follicular cells into lutein cells   **20.10**

(c) **F** The corpus luteum is an important source of progesterone during early pregnancy (i.e. before placental production is established). In the non-pregnant state the ovary does produce oestradiol but in pregnancy the placenta becomes the main site of production   **20.11**

(d) **F** Progesterone antagonizes the renal sodium-retaining effects of mineralocorticoids. In pregnancy, the high progesterone levels and their consequent renal effects lead to a secondary elevation in plasma aldosterone levels   **20.11**

(e) **F** The hepatic metabolism of progesterone is so rapid that in low doses it is ineffective when taken orally. Synthetic derivatives of testosterone and progesterone are active orally and are used as contraceptives and in treating menstrual disorders   **20.11**

A211 (a) **F** Progesterone is produced by the corpus luteum following ovulation   **20.10**

(b) **T** This change is necessary for acceptance of the fertilized egg and subsequent implantation of the embryo   **20.11**

(c) **F** Progesterone suppresses this response; it is oestrogen that enhances it   **20.11**

(d) **T** Maintained production of progesterone increases the weight of the uterus and its nucleic acid, collagen, glycogen and lipid contents, and stimulates development of the secretory alveoli of the mammary gland   **20.11**

(e) **T** The principal metabolites are pregnanolone, pregnanediol and allopregnanediol   **20.11**

Q212 In the human female:

(a) hydroxylation of progesterone gives rise only to compounds with progestogenic effects

(b) prolonged use of exogenous oestrogens causes muscle wasting

(c) all endogenous oestrogens are synthesized from androgen precursors

(d) oestradiol appears in large amounts in the urine

(e) exogenous oestrogens may cause oedema

Q213 Oestrogens:

(a) are mainly produced in the developing follicles in non-pregnant women

(b) produced by the placenta in pregnancy are largely in the form of oestradiol

(c) can both stimulate and inhibit lactation

(d) act by binding to the target tissues

(e) act by stimulating adenylate cyclase activity and the production of cyclic AMP

A212 (a) **F** Hydroxylation of progesterone also gives rise to precursors of androgens, glucocorticoids and mineralocorticoids   **20.11**

(b) **F** Oestrogens have an anabolic effect (albeit less than that of androgens), i.e. they cause retention of nitrogen, phosphate and potassium. They act in opposition to glucocorticoids reducing protein catabolism and breakdown of amino acids   **20.14**

(c) **T** Although oestradiol may be converted into oestrone (and vice versa) and oestriol may be produced from oestradiol or oestrone (via 16α-hydroxyoestrone) these compounds are all synthesized from androgen precursors derived from cholesterol   **20.14**

(d) **F** Oestradiol is strongly bound to a specific transport protein in the plasma and hence is not freely filtered. It is mainly metabolized by the liver, and the glucuronide and sulphate derivatives are excreted in the urine and faeces   **20.15**

(e) **T** Unlike progesterone, oestrogens cause sodium, and hence, fluid retention. The increase in ECF volume may cause oedema and, if severe, may precipitate cardiac failure   **20.18**

A213 (a) **T** The cells of the theca interna and stratum granulosum produce oestrogens   **20.10, 20.14**

(b) **F** The placenta produces increasing amounts of oestriol; oestradiol and oestrone are the primary products of ovarian secretion   **20.15**

(c) **T** Oestrogens can act with prolactin to stimulate and maintain lactation, but at high doses oestrogens inhibit lactation   **20.14, 20.60**

(d) **T** There are two binding components, one nuclear and one cytosolic; there is a strong affinity for oestrogen binding by the cytosolic component   **20.16**

(e) **F** The bound oestrogen complex stimulates RNA synthesis, and hence protein synthesis, within the target tissue   **20.16**

Q214 Considering gonadotrophic hormones:

    (a)   FSH in the male increases androgen production

    (b)   FSH levels may be high in postmenopausal females

    (c)   FSH levels may be high in castrated males

    (d)   LH alone is responsible for maintaining production of progesterone during early pregnancy

    (e)   human chorionic gonadotrophin may be used in the treatment of sickle-cell anaemia

Q215 In the human menstrual cycle:

    (a)   the stratum basalis of the endometrium proliferates between the end of menstruation and the day of ovulation

    (b)   ovulation is preceded by a sharp rise in release of oestradiol

    (c)   LH stimulates the production of progesterone from the corpus luteum following ovulation

    (d)   a fall in oestradiol secretion is necessary to promote menstruation

    (e)   body temperature rises just prior to ovulation

A214	(a)	F	FSH in the male stimulates and maintains spermato-genesis by promoting the development of the germinal epithelium of the seminiferous tubules, but it has no effect on androgen production by Leydig cells	20.19
	(b)	T	Presumably because the negative feedback effects of oestrogens on the hypothalamus are lost and FSH secretion from the adenohypophysis is disinhibited (oestrogen treatment causes a fall in FSH)	20.19
	(c)	F	In the male ICSH (which appears to be identical to LH) is elevated in the absence of androgenic feedback inhibiting the hypothalamic releasing factor	20.19
	(d)	F	LH together with FSH promotes the formation of the corpus luteum and progesterone biosynthesis. Furthermore, chorionic cells of the placenta produce an LH-like hormone (chorionic gonadotrophin) that acts to maintain progesterone production	20.19
	(e)	T	Human chorionic gonadotrophin stimulates the synthesis of fetal haemoglobin (haemoglobin F, $\alpha_2^F\gamma_2^F$); since the sickling trait is due to a 6-valine variant of the normal 6-glutamine β chain, the elevated levels of fetal haemoglobin may mask the abnormality	20.20
A215	(a)	F	During this period (proliferative phase) the stratum *functionalis* regenerates	20.21
	(b)	T	This renders the endometrium 'oestrogen-primed' (i.e. responsive to progesterone) for the next phase of the cycle	20.21
	(c)	T	The progesterone transforms the endometrium into a secretory endothelium in preparation for acceptance of the fertilized egg	20.21, 20.11
	(d)	F	Normally, both progesterone and oestradiol secretion rates fall at the end of the menstrual cycle and menstruation occurs. If progesterone levels are maintained, menstruation does not occur	20.21
	(e)	F	The temperature rise (about 0.5 °C) occurs just after ovulation and is due to increased progesterone levels	20.21

Q216 Considering the menstrual cycle:

(a) the menopause occurs when FSH is no longer secreted in sufficient amounts

(b) there is a surge of progesterone just before ovulation

(c) there is a surge of oestradiol just before ovulation

(d) sodium retention by the kidneys often occurs during the last week

(e) after ovulation the endometrium rapidy degenerates

Q217 During sexual intercourse:

(a) increased activity in sacral parasympathetic nerves causes the erectile tissue in the penis to become engorged with blood

(b) vaginal stimulation causes release of oxytocin

(c) ejaculation is produced by smooth muscle contraction at the root of the penis

(d) impairment of the parasympathetic innervation causes failure of ejaculation

(e) orgasm in the female is normally preceded by rapid respiration

A216 (a) **F**   Menopausal women have high circulating FSH levels;   **20.21**
the menopause usually occurs between 40 to 50 years
when the primordial follicles are exhausted (hence there
is no 'end organ' for the action of FSH)

     (b) **F**   Progesterone is synthesized by the corpus luteum (a   **20.21**
structure derived from follicular cells after ovulation)
under the influence of LH and FSH

     (c) **T**   Oestradiol is produced by the follicular cells of the devel-   **20.21**
oping ovum under the influence of FSH and LH. FSH
levels are high during the early part of the cycle and
oestradiol synthesis is induced

     (d) **T**   As the levels of progesterone fall, its antimineralocorti-   **20.21**
coid effect wanes and this occurs against a background
of elevated aldosterone levels (the system having been
activated to oppose the natriuretic effects of progesterone)

     (e) **F**   The 'oestrogen-primed' endometrium is acted upon by   **20.21**
progesterone (synthesized by the corpus luteum) and
goes into the secretory phase during which the glandular
pits begin to secrete and the vasculature becomes more
extensive (in preparation for implantation)

A217 (a) **T**   Parasympathetically mediated vasodilatation causes   **20.24**
increased arterial blood flow; a rise in pressure com-
presses the veins and the erectile tissue becomes
engorged with blood

     (b) **T**   Vaginal stimulation elicits reflex release of oxytocin   **20.24**
from the posterior pituitary; this promotes uterine con-
tractions and thus facilitates transport of seminal fluid

     (c) **F**   Rhythmic contractions of striated muscles which com-   **20.24**
press the urethra at the root of the penis are largely res-
ponsible for ejaculation

     (d) **F**   Sympathetic impairment leads to failure of ejaculation.   **20.24**
This problem is encountered as a side-effect of treat-
ment with noradrenergic neurone blocking drugs, α
methyldopa, etc

     (e) **F**   In the male, pre-orgasmic respiration is rapid and   **20.24**
shallow. In the female there are commonly periods of
breath-holding before orgasm

Q218 In human semen:

(a) spermatozoa comprise about 10% of the seminal volume

(b) citric acid in the seminal plasma is derived from the seminal vesicles

(c) the anterior cap of the spermatozoa is a lysosome

(d) sperm motility is achieved by movement of the tail-piece only

(e) the process of activation of acrosomal enzymes is known as decapacitation

Q219 The process of fertilization of the ovum:

(a) takes place only within the Fallopian tube

(b) is facilitated by progesterone

(c) is species specific

(d) results in identical twins being produced if two ova are released and fertilized at the same time

(e) is impaired by the carbonic anhydrase inhibitor, acetazolamide

Q220 After fertilization of the ovum:

(a) mitotic division begins during passage down the Fallopian tube

(b) endometrial hypertrophy begins when the blastocyst reaches the uterus

(c) the trophoblast cells are responsible for implantation (nidation)

(d) the corpus luteum is maintained by progesterone

(e) the embryonic knot develops as an accumulation of cells at one pole of the blastocyst

A218	(a)	T	Ejaculated volume is approximately 3 ml in which there are 200–600 million spermatozoa	20.24
	(b)	F	Fructose, inositol and sorbitol are derived from the seminal vesicles; citric acid is contained in the prostatic secretion	20.24
	(c)	T	This is termed the acrosome. It contains hyaluronidase and an enzyme complex which breaks down the outer layers of the ovum	20.25, 2.12
	(d)	F	The middle piece is also involved in movement; both have the 9:2 arrangement of coarse and fine fibrils seen in flagellae	20.25
	(e)	F	This process (which involves removal of a decapacitation factor) is known as capacitation	20.25

A219	(a)	T	For this reason and since the ovum is only in the Fallopian tube for a few days, the mating process only results in fertilization during these days	20.25
	(b)	F	Progesterone reduces the activity of Fallopian tubular secretions which normally operate to denude the ovum of its corona radiata; progesterone also inhibits capacitation	20.25, 20.26
	(c)	T	This may be due to the presence of protein (*fertilizin*) on the ovum which reacts with an anti-fertilizin on the sperm of the same species only	20.26
	(d)	F	This results in dizygotic (non-identical) twins. Identical twins are the result of separation of the two blastomeres which each then develop and implant	20.26
	(e)	T	This is because bicarbonate ions are involved in the process of denudation of the ovum	20.26

A220	(a)	T	The time taken for the fertilized egg to reach the uterus is about 5 days, by which time it has reached the blastocyst stage	20.26
	(b)	F	This process starts at ovulation, under the influence of progesterone from the corpus luteum	20.26
	(c)	T	These cells grow into projections (chorionic villi) which penetrate the endometrium	20.26
	(d)	F	Some chorionic cells secrete chorionic gonadotrophin which maintains the corpus luteum and thus sustains progesterone secretion	20.26
	(e)	T	This is the primordium of the fetus	20.26

Q221 In the female, following sexual intercourse:

 (a) fertilization may be impaired by the carbonic anhydrase inhibitor, acetazolamide

 (b) implantation may be jeopardized by noradrenergic neurone blocking drugs

 (c) fertilization may be impaired by the anti-oestrogen clomiphene

 (d) fertilization may be impaired by acid media in the cervical canal

 (e) fertilization is most efficiently suppressed by an intrauterine device (IUD)

Q222 Synthetic oestrogens:

 (a) may be used to alleviate dysmenorrhoea (painful menstruation)

 (b) may be used to treat female infertility

 (c) may be used as postcoital contraceptives

 (d) may cause thromboembolism

 (e) are used to promote lactation

A221 (a) **T** Fallopian tube secretions play a role in the process of   **20.26**
fertilization by attacking the corona radiata from the
ovum and facilitating sperm penetration. Since bicarbonate ions in the Fallopian secretions influence the
effectiveness of denudation, carbonic anhydrase inhibitors impair this process

   (b) **T** An increase in the delay between fertilization and the   **20.26**
arrival of the blastocyst in the uterus may adversely
affect implantation. Peristaltic activity of tubular
smooth muscle is augmented by its noradrenergic innervation, thus interference with this may impair implantation

   (c) **F** Clomiphene inhibits the interaction of oestradiol with   **20.27**
oestrogen receptors and hence suppresses the feedback
inhibition of pituitary gonadotrophin secretion by the
hypothalamus. Given during the fifth to tenth day of the
menstrual cycle it usually induces ovulation

   (d) **T** Acid media reduce the viability of spermatozoa (seminal   **20.3**
plasma is alkaline) and render them more susceptible to
spermicidal agents. Spermicidal agents often contain a
material that physically impairs sperm motility, a
material toxic to sperm and a compound that renders the
preparation acidic

   (e) **F** The most effective contraception is achieved with oral   **20.29**
contraceptives (about 4% failure rate — largely due to
non-compliance). IUDs have a failure rate of 7% compared to intravaginal spermicides with a failure rate of
about 27%

A222 (a) **T** They suppress ovulation and hence the normal endo-   **20.22**
metrial changes induced by progesterone (the pain is
thought to be due to prostaglandins secreted by the endometrium)

   (b) **F** Anti-oestrogens are used in this disorder; they prevent   **20.18,**
the feedback inhibition of oestradiol on to the anterior   **20.17**
pituitary and hence permit gonadotrophin release

   (c) **T** The antifertility effect is thought to be due to decreased   **20.34**
transit time of the fertilized egg through the Fallopian
tube giving insufficient time for development

   (d) **T** This is due to a combination of increased coagulation   **20.40**
factors VII and X, increased platelet aggregation and
decreased fibrinolytic activity

   (e) **F** Oestrogen inhibits prolactin secretion and hence milk   **20.60**
production

Q223 Oral contraceptive preparations:

(a) containing oestrogen and progesterone are the most effective

(b) containing progesterone only may be advantageous after childbirth

(c) may lead to iron-deficiency anaemia

(d) may be lead to hypertension

(e) may be used to treat excessive menstrual bleeding

Q224 Combined oestrogen–progesterone preparations:

(a) are used as contraceptives because they inhibit LH release

(b) alter the properties of the cervical mucosa to hinder passage of spermatozoa

(c) inhibit endogenous oestrogen production

(d) may alleviate headaches

(e) shorten the period of endometrial proliferation and secretion

Q225 During gestation:

(a) ectoderm cells surround the amniotic cavity and endoderm cells surround the yolk sac

(b) mesoderm cells are found between the ectoderm and endoderm only

(c) umbilical blood vessels arise from endoderm cells

(d) primordial sex glands appear in the fourth week

(e) sexual differentiation is partly determined by the level of fetal oestrogens

A223 (a) **T** The progesterone modifies cervical secretory activity such that movement of spermatozoa through it is less easy and the endometrium is less receptive to the fertilized ovum. The oestrogen inhibits follicular development by suppressing FSH release 20.30

(b) **T** This is because the other products contain oestrogens which suppress lactation 20.33

(c) **F** Although a reduction in plasma vitamin B_{12} may predispose users of oral contraceptives to macrocytic anaemia, the incidence of iron-deficiency anaemia is lower, presumably due to reduced menstrual blood loss 20.33

(d) **T** There are several possible explanations for this; the most popular hypothesis is that the hypertension is due to stimulation of the renin–angiotensin–aldosterone axis 20.34

(e) **T** Excessive bleeding is usually due to impaired progesterone production of the corpus luteum 20.22

A224 (a) **F** Much higher doses than are used as contraceptives do inhibit LH release; the contraceptive effect of the oestrogen is through inhibiting FSH release 20.31

(b) **T** This is an effect of the progestogen component; the cervical secretion becomes scanty and the mucus loses its properties 20.21

(c) **T** This is because follicle development is impaired 20.31

(d) **F** Oral contraceptives aggravate symptoms in women predisposed to premenstrual migrainous headache 20.34

(e) **T** There may be a considerable diminution in the cyclical changes in the stratum functionalis — this provides a further anti-fertility effect by rendering the endometrium less favourable for implantation 20.31

A225 (a) **T** Ectodermal cells form the amniotic membrane; the cells in the region where the amniotic cavity and yolk sac are juxtaposed form the embryonic disc (from this the body of the embryo develops) 20.36

(b) **F** A layer of mesoderm cells also develops adjacent to the trophoblast cells to form a double membrane — the chorion 20.37

(c) **F** The two umbilical arteries and one umbilical vein develop from the mesoderm 20.37

(d) **T** These are formed from ectodermal and mesodermal tissue. Germ cells then migrate into the glands and the glands differentiate in the seventh week 20.38

(e) **F** The synthesis of androgens by fetal Leydig cells determines sexual differentiation; in their absence the female course of development ensues 20.38

Q226 In the fetal circulation:

    (a)   most of the blood delivered to the left atrium comes from the pulmonary circulation

    (b)   blood from the right ventricle joins blood from the left ventricle in the aorta

    (c)   the oxygen saturation of blood in the umbilical vein is less than that in umbilical arteries

    (d)   the foramen ovale normally closes at birth

    (e)   the ductus venosus joins the inferior vena cava

Q227 In the cardiovascular system of the pre-term fetus:

    (a)   blood flows from the placenta into the fetal circulation via the umbilical arteries

    (b)   the ductus venosus provides a route by which umbilical venous blood may by-pass the fetal liver

    (c)   maternal blood passes into the fetal circulation via the placenta

    (d)   blood is shunted from left to right atrium through the foramen ovale

    (e)   approximately half the fetal cardiac output does not pass through fetal capillaries

A226 (a) **F** Blood delivered to the left atrium comes mostly from the right atrium through the foramen ovale in the interatrial septum   **20.38**

(b) **T** This occurs through an opening known as the ductus arteriosus   **20.38**

(c) **F** The blood in the umbilical vein (transporting blood to the fetus) has an oxygen saturation of about 55–70%; that in the umbilical artery is about 25–40% saturated   **20.39**

(d) **T** This is due to high pressure in the left atrium as a result of the initial respiratory movements increasing the return of blood in the pulmonary veins   **20.39**

(e) **T** This contains the most oxygenated, and nutritionally rich blood, travelling from the umbilical vein towards the heart   **20.39**

A227 (a) **F** Blood returns to the placenta via the umbilical arteries and re-enters the fetal circulation via the umbilical vein   **20.39**

(b) **T** Thus a significant fraction of relatively well-oxygenated blood may return to the heart without passage through hepatic capillaries   **20.39**

(c) **F** The placenta is an organ in which small molecules are exchanged between maternal and fetal blood via the chorionic villi, but whole blood does not cross the placental barrier   **20.39**

(d) **F** Right atrial pressue is slightly greater than left atrial pressure throughout the cardiac cycle because the volume of blood entering the right atrium via the venae cavae is much greater than pulmonary venous return to the left atrium, hence the shunt through the foramen ovale is from right to left   **20.38**

(e) **T** This large fraction of the cardiac output therefore does not exchange oxygen with the tissues and thus provides an important buffer against desaturation of haemoglobin   **20.38**

Q228 In the circulation of a healthy fetus at birth:

    (a)   lung inflation causes pulmonary vasoconstriction

    (b)   the ductus arteriosus begins to constrict

    (c)   the venous return of blood to the left atrium is increased

    (d)   the increase in right atrial pressure closes the foramen ovale

    (e)   the smooth muscle of the umbilical vessels constricts

Q229 During pregnancy:

    (a)   transplacental oxygen exchange is entirely passive

    (b)   the placenta provides a barrier to the passage of all exogenous substances into the fetus

    (c)   human chorionic somatomammotrophin (HCS) enhances insulin secretion

    (d)   human chorionic somatomammotrophin (HCS) is an important determinant of fetal growth

    (e)   the placenta contains high levels of choline acetyltransferase and acetylcholinesterase

A228 (a) **F** Lung inflation causes pulmonary vasodilatation, increasing pulmonary blood flow and initiating gas exchange between pulmonary blood and alveolar air 20.39

(b) **T** The mechanism is not identified. Closure of the ductus arteriosus reduces, and then arrests the shunting of right ventricular blood into the systemic arterial circulation 20.38

(c) **T** The increase in pulmonary blood flow (see (a)) increases pulmonary venous return 20.39

(d) **F** The reduced venous return to the right atrium together with the increased pulmonary venous return reverses the pressure gradient across the interatrial septum. This closes the foramen ovale because of the structure of septum primum and septum secundum which constitute the foramen 20.39

(e) **T** Possibly due to catecholamines, trauma, hypoxaemia or a combination of these and other factors there is powerful contraction of the smooth muscle which can occlude the vessels 20.39

A229 (a) **F** Although diffusion of oxygen from maternal to fetal blood is partly passive (and facilitated by the great affinity for oxygen of fetal haemoglobin) there is also active oxygen transport (a process involving placental cytochrome — P_{450}) 20.40

(b) **F** Although the placenta does offer a barrier to movement of many substances from mother to fetus, numerous drugs (particularly lipophilic molecules) readily cross 20.40

(c) **F** HCS inhibits the action of insulin (by suppressing its secretion) and hence causes a reduction in maternal uptake of glucose and amino acids. While this may be beneficial to the fetus it probably explains the worsening condition of patients with diabetes mellitus during pregnancy 20.40

(d) **F** Although HCS is growth-hormone-like (and cross-reacts with antibodies to the latter) its effects are largely confined to stimulating development of the mother's breasts. Furthermore, little HCS crosses the placenta to reach the fetus 20.40

(e) **T** Although not innervated by cholinergic nerves, the placenta contains very high levels of these enzymes and many more (MAO, COMT, renin, etc.). They are probably involved in deactivating circulating substances or in local synthesis 20.41

Q230 The human placenta:

(a) permits passage of nutrients and waste products
(b) produces only two hormones, oestriol and progesterone
(c) produces a substance which promotes breast development
(d) increases its secretion of oestrogens towards the end of pregnancy
(e) suppresses ovarian follicle development

Q231 During labour:

(a) maternal adrenal steroids inhibit progesterone production
(b) fetal corticosteroids increase prostaglandin synthesis in the placenta
(c) the responsiveness of the myometrium to the contractile effect of oxytocin increases
(d) uterine contractions initially have a frequency of about one per minute
(e) intrauterine pressure can rise to about 100 mmHg during expulsion

Q232 Lactation (milk production):

(a) is initiated by a fall in oestrogen production at birth
(b) is maintained by suckling
(c) is enhanced by oxytocin
(d) is inhibited by dopamine-like drugs
(e) results in milk secretion when the myoepithelial cells of the alveolar ducts are stimulated by catecholamines

A230 (a) **T** Passive movements are believed to be assisted by active transport   **20.40**

(b) **F** Chorionic gonadotrophin and chorionic somatomammotrophin are also produced   **20.40**

(c) **T** This is the function of chorionic somatomammotrophin   **20.40**

(d) **T** The functions of the oestrogens are to promote myometrial growth, alter the cervix in such a way as to facilitate dilatation and to enhance haemostatic mechanisms   **20.40**

(e) **T** It does this by secreting large amounts of oestrogen and progesterone, which act on the hypothalamus to inhibit release of FSH and LH   **20.41**

A231 (a) **F** It is cortisol from the fetal adrenal gland which inhibits placental progesterone production   **20.53**

(b) **T** Prostaglandin $F_{2\alpha}$ production is increased, which further inhibits progesterone secretion and stimulates oestrogen synthesis   **12.36, 25.53**

(c) **T** This is due to the increased oestrogen production and reduced progesterone secretion   **20.54**

(d) **F** During the first stage of labour the frequency of uterine contractions is about 1–4 per hour   **20.53**

(e) **T** This rise in pressure may facilitate further rhythmic contractions during delivery   **20.53, 20.54**

A232 (a) **T** This removes the inhibitory influence on the anterior pituitary thus permitting prolactin release   **20.60**

(b) **T** Nipple stimulation elicits a reflex increase in prolactin release   **20.60**

(c) **F** Oxytocin facilitates milk secretion — not production   **20.60**

(d) **T** Drugs such as bromocriptine mimic the suppressive effect of dopamine on prolactin release   **20.61, 19.10**

(e) **F** Catecholamines or sympathetic stimulation cause the myoepithelial cells to relax and thereby inhibit milk secretion   **20.60**

Central Nervous System

Q233 In the central nervous system of man:

(a) neuroglial cells are non-neuronal
(b) the term funiculus may be applied to a group of cell bodies
(c) microglial cells are principally concerned with the transport of nutrients and metabolites between the neurones and the blood stream
(d) the term nucleus may be applied to a group of associated cell bodies
(e) the maximal degree of myelination occurs at the completion of postnatal growth (about 17 years)

Q234 In the spinal cord:

(a) the white matter is mainly composed of myelinated and non-myelinated fibres
(b) fibres said to be conducting impulses 'rostrally' carry information in a proximo-distal direction
(c) interneurones lie entirely within the white matter
(d) cell bodies in the lateral horns of the grey matter give rise to the preganglionic fibres of the autonomic nervous system
(e) the posterior horns of the grey matter contain the cell bodies of the afferent fibres of the spinal nerves

Q235 In normal healthy man, cerebrospinal fluid (CSF):

(a) has the same composition as plasma
(b) has a slightly higher pH than that of plasma
(c) is produced at a rate of about 0.3 ml/min
(d) pressure is about 20 mmHg in the supine position
(e) has a high buffering capacity

A233 (a) **T** There are three types of neuroglial cells — astrocytes (concerned with provision of nutrients, etc.); oligodendrocytes (concerned with the formation of myelin), and microglia (a type of macrophage)   6.1

(b) **F** Funiculus (little cord) may be applied to groups of nerve fibres   6.1

(c) **F** This is the function of the astrocytes (see (a))   6.1

(d) **T** Nucleus, ganglion, body or corpus are all used in this context   6.1

(e) **T** All nerve fibres initially lack a myelin sheath — the onset of their functional activity coincides with the laying down of myelin   6.4

A234 (a) **T** The white matter almost surrounds an H-shaped mass of grey matter (where the cell bodies are found)   6.4

(b) **F** Rostral (towards the beak), cranial or cephalic all refer to ascending fibres; descending tracts convey impulses *caudally*   6.4

(c) **F** These neurones may relay information from sensory to motor fibres within the cord; they lie in the grey matter   6.4

(d) **T** These are located in the lateral horns (intermediolateral columns) of the thoracic and the upper two or three lumbar segments — they leave the cord in the anterior roots   6.4, 9.1–2

(e) **F** These cell bodies lie outside the spinal cord in the dorsal (posterior) root ganglion; in the posterior horns the afferent fibres synapse with interneurones or neurones of ascending tracts   6.2

A235 (a) **F** It contains very little protein, has lower potassium, calcium and phosphate concentrations and higher chloride concentrations   6.12

(b) **F** CSF is slightly more acidic than plasma — by about 0.1 pH unit   6.12

(c) **T** The components are mostly actively secreted from the choroid plexuses lining the lateral and third ventricles — the total volume is about 200 ml   6.12

(d) **F** When lying down, CSF pressure is about 10 cm of CSF in the lumbar cistern; when sitting it is about 30 cm of CSF   6.12

(e) **F** The buffering capacity of CSF is low; an acute rise of CSF P_{CO_2} by 1 mmHg increases the $[H^+]$ by 4–5 nmol/l whereas in blood, a similar change increases $[H^+]$ by about 0.8 nmol/l   28.20

Q236 In normal man, cerebrospinal fluid:

   (a)   is formed at a rate of about 3 ml/min
   (b)   has a higher K^+ concentration than plasma
   (c)   pressure is about 40 mmHg in the lateral recumbent position
   (d)   has a colloid osmotic pressure of about 25 mmHg
   (e)   is most safely sampled from the cisterna magna

Q237 The passage of substances from the peripheral blood into the brain:

   (a)   is hindered by the presence of astrocytes
   (b)   is less likely to occur if the substance is strongly protein-bound
   (c)   is more likely to occur if the substance is lipid soluble
   (d)   is not influenced by the plasma pH
   (e)   may occur more rapidly than normal in certain disease states

Q238 In man, the penetration of a substance into the brain from the blood:

   (a)   is affected by the affinity with which it binds to plasma proteins
   (b)   is affected by the degree to which it is ionized at plasma pH
   (c)   is affected by its lipid–water partition coefficient
   (d)   is low in the region of the hypothalamus
   (e)   may be reduced in meningitis

A236 (a) **F**   It is formed at a rate of about 0.3 ml/min, both by passive diffusion and active secretion (mainly by the choroid plexuses associated with the lateral and third ventricles)   6.12

     (b) **F**   CSF potassium concentration is usually 2–3 mmol/l compared to 3.8–5 mmol/l for plasma; this indicates there is an active extrusion of K^+ from cerebrospinal fluid — probably to regulate the level and hence prevent interference with neuronal functions   6.12

     (c) **F**   In the lateral recumbent position in the lumbar cistern the CSF pressure is 10–15 cm of CSF; sitting, the pressure is 30–40 cm of CSF   6.12

     (d) **F**   CSF contains very little protein (0.2–0.4 g/kg compared to 60–80 g/kg for plasma) and hence has a negligible colloid osmotic pressure   6.12

     (e) **F**   The safest sampling site is from the lumbar cistern where the spinal column contains only subarachnoid space and spinal nerves   6.12

A237 (a) **T**   The astrocytes (and their processes) which cover the walls of a large percentage (85%) of the capillaries provide a second barrier through which a substance needs to pass   6.12

     (b) **T**   Brain interstitial fluid is virtually free of protein. Substances bound tightly to plasma proteins do not enter since these proteins do not pass into the CSF   6.12

     (c) **T**   There is good correlation between rate of penetration and lipid solubility   6.13

     (d) **F**   The degree of ionization influences the ability of substances to cross the blood–brain barrier and this will be influenced by changes in pH   6.13

     (e) **T**   Hypertension and meningitis are conditions in which the 'blood–brain barrier' may become leaky   6.13

A238 (a) **T**   Protein is largely excluded from brain interstitial fluid and CSF   6.12

     (b) **T**   The lipid-soluble, non-ionized substances penetrate more readily   6.12

     (c) **T**   Greater lipid solubility enhances penetration   6.13

     (d) **F**   The posterior pituitary and the adjacent parts of the hypothalamus are outside the 'blood–brain barrier', have a rich blood supply and are, therefore, readily accessible   6.13

     (e) **F**   Meningitis tends to disrupt the 'blood–brain barrier' and hence substances more readily gain access to the central nervous system   6.13

Q239 Sensory receptors:

(a) which are tonically active, provide information about changes in stimulus strength

(b) showing marked adaptation provide information about the rate of change of stimulus strength

(c) transmit information about the strength of the stimulus by variations in the amplitudes of the action potentials generated

(d) described as thermoreceptors respond equally to rises and falls in temperature

(e) mediating different sensations do so because of their central connections

Q240 Sensory receptors:

(a) responsive to mechanical distortion may have free or encapsulated nerve endings

(b) always adapt to a continuously applied stimulus

(c) which show a tonic discharge rapidly adapt to a continuous stimulus

(d) responsive to temperature have myelinated and unmyelinated afferents

(e) located near the medullary respiratory centres on the ventral surface of the brain respond directly to changes in CO_2

A239 (a) **F**   Tonic receptors discharge continuously in response to a   **6.14**
stimulus of fixed strength, and thus provide continuous
information about the status of the body

(b) **T**   Such phasic receptors do not transmit a continuous   **6.14**
signal, but signal most strongly when the stimulus
changes

(c) **F**   The action potentials generated are of a fixed amplitude;   **6.14**
the strength of the signal is coded in the frequency of discharge of action potentials (and in the number of nerve
fibres activated)

(d) **F**   There are warm thermoreceptors and cold thermorecep-   **31.7**
tors; they are differentially sensitive to rises or falls in
temperature and have different thresholds

(e) **T**   All sensory nerve fibres convey information through   **6.14**
action potential discharges; thus the sensation evoked is
due to the specific central projections of these afferent
fibres

A240 (a) **T**   There are many different types of mechanoreceptors   **6.14**
some of which are close to the surface and some of which
are more deeply situated; the endings may be free,
encapsulated or specialized (e.g. Golgi tendon organs)

(b) **T**   This adaptation may be partial or complete, and either   **6.14**
slow or rapid

(c) **F**   Tonic receptors adapt poorly and slowly; they continue   **6.14**
to inform the brain of the status of the body

(d) **T**   Thermoreceptors are associated with fine, myelinated A   **31.7**
fibres and non-myelinated C fibres which ascend the
spinal cord and relay in the thalamus

(e) **F**   An increase in arterial P_{CO_2} does result in stimulation of   **24.10**
these receptors but it is through the production of H^+
$(CO_2 + H_2O \rightleftharpoons H_2CO_3 \rightleftharpoons H^+ + HCO_3^-)$

Q241 Pain:

(a) perceived as a diffuse sensation is transmitted by myelinated A fibres

(b) perception is mediated by cells in the substantia gelatinosa that receive an excitatory input from the Aδ and C fibres from pain receptors

(c) sensation is abolished if the cerebral cortex is removed

(d) sensations arising from viscera are often sensed at a site away from the origin of the stimulus

(e) sensations are transmitted to higher centres in the anterolateral columns

Q242 The sensation of pain:

(a) may be transmitted by first-order neurones that are myelinated and conduct at 12–30 m/s

(b) may be transmitted by first-order neurones that are unmyelinated and conduct at 0.5–2 m/s

(c) may be influenced by higher centres modulating neurotransmission at the level of the substantia gelatinosa

(d) may be reduced by endogenous substances such as kinins and prostaglandins

(e) due to excitation of visceral afferents is precisely localized

Q243 In the human ear:

(a) the auditory ossicles lie in a fluid-filled cavity

(b) the stapes fits into an oval window in the wall of the inner ear

(c) the inner ear contains a fluid-filled spiral canal which is divided into two compartments

(d) the perception of sound is achieved by mechanical deformation of hair processes in the organ of Corti

(e) the frequency of nerve impulses in the cochlear nerve is directly related to the frequency of sound waves

A241 (a) **F** Two types of fibre transmit pain — Aδ fibres (fast-conducting, myelinated) are responsible for immediate 'fast' pain, whilst C fibres (slower-conducting, unmyelinated) are responsible for the duller, aching, more diffuse pain **6.16**

(b) **F** The Aδ fibres excite, whereas the C fibres inhibit neurones in the substantia gelatinosa **6.16**

(c) **F** Although the cortex does influence the perception of pain, the thalamus is the main region for integration of the input **6.17**

(d) **T** This is known as referred pain and probably arises because the sensory neurones from the visceral organ and those from the region to which the pain is referred form synapses with the same second-order neurones **6.17**

(e) **T** Decussation occurs at the spinal level, and the axons of the second-order neurones travel in the anterolateral columns and synapse in the thalamus **6.15**

A242 (a) **T** These fibres fall into the Aδ (i.e. Group III) category and are responsible for the rapid appreciation of a painful stimulus **6.16**

(b) **T** These are C (i.e. Group IV) fibres and are responsible for the slower appreciation of the more diffuse pain evoked by a noxious stimulus **6.16**

(c) **T** Higher centres may have excitatory or inhibitory effects on cells in the substantia gelatinosa that modify transmission of afferent information **6.16**

(d) **F** Inflammatory processes produce kinins and prostaglandins; these substances depolarize pain endings and thus make them more excitable **6.16**

(e) **F** Visceral pain is often referred to the body surface or to a structure that developed from the same embryonic segment as the viscus affected **6.16**

A243 (a) **F** The ossicles (malleus, incus, stapes) are in an air-filled cavity which is connected to the pharynx by the Eustachian tube; this serves to equalize the pressure on either side of the eardrum **6.18**

(b) **T** It is across this oval window that the sound waves are transmitted from middle to inner ear **6.18, 6.19**

(c) **F** The spiral canal (cochlea) is divided into three compartments, all of which are fluid filled **6.18**

(d) **T** Movement of fluid against the hair processes deforms them and gives rise to impulses in the cochlear nerve **6.19**

(e) **F** The frequency of impulses is determined by the loudness of the signal — weak tones set up a low frequency, loud tones a high frequency **6.19**

Q244 Considering the vestibular system of a human subject:

(a) rotation about the vertical axis is detected by the horizontal (lateral) semicircular canals

(b) endolymph moving away from an ampulla causes its sensory nerves to discharge

(c) rotation to the right (about the vertical axis) is initially accompanied by nystagmus in the opposite direction

(d) the functioning of the superior semicircular canals can be tested by irrigating the external auditory meatus with water at 30 °C

(e) stimulation of its sensory nerves influences activity in α motor neurones

Q245 The reticular formation:

(a) regulates the tone of skeletal muscles

(b) determines the level of consciousness via ascending fibres passing to the cortex

(c) is not influenced by cortical activity

(d) is responsible for initiating the conscious desire to sleep

(e) is sensitive to metabolic influences

A244 (a) **T** With the head tilted 30° forward, these canals are at 6.19 right angles to the vertical. Rotation about the vertical axis thus more effectively stimulates the horizontal than the superior or posterior canals

(b) **F** Endolymph moving away from an ampulla unloads the 6.19 cupola and causes an inhibition of sensory nerve discharge. Endolymph moving towards the ampulla displaces the cupola and hence stimulates its sensory endings

(c) **F** At the onset of rotation the left ampulla is stimulated and 6.19 the right ampulla is unloaded. This results in a slow movement of the eyes to the left followed by a quick flick to the right (nystagmus to the right)

(d) **F** In a supine subject with head raised 30° from the horizontal, the competence of the lateral (horizontal) semicircular canals can be tested in this way. The water cools the endolymph, rendering it more dense; it moves (under the force of gravity) towards the ampulla on the irrigated side. The superior semicircular canals are not stimulated by this manoeuvre 6.19

(e) **T** There are connections between the vestibular system 6.20 and the cerebellum, the neurones innervating the extraocular muscles, and, via the vestibulospinal tracts, α motor neurones in the ventral horns. This pathway subserves adjustments of tone in postural muscles

A245 (a) **T** It receives an input from the cerebellum, basal ganglia 6.22 and the muscles themselves; fibres pass from the reticular formation down the cord in the reticulospinal tracts and synapse with lower motor neurones and cell bodies of γ motor neurones

(b) **T** These fibres end, mainly, in the frontal lobes of the 6.22 cortex; they influence all sensory and mentational activities of the cortex

(c) **F** There is a feedback mechanism whereby ascending 6.22 fibres from the reticular formation are influenced by the cortex — this is probably responsible for sudden shifts in attention and alertness in response to a novel stimulus

(d) **F** This arises from inhibitory signals in descending fibres 6.23 from the cortex to the reticular activating system

(e) **T** It is also influenced by many drugs; such effects lead to 6.23 changes in the level of consciousness and behaviour

Q246 In normal man:

(a) the intake of food is partly governed by the level of blood glucose

(b) an increase in body fluid osmolality stimulates thirst

(c) the dominant rhythm of the EEG during wakefulness is the α rhythm (frequency 8–13 Hz)

(d) the reticular formation becomes activated during REM (rapid eye movement) sleep

(e) the dominant rhythm of the EEG during non REM sleep is the δ rhythm (1–8 Hz)

Q247 With maintained administration, some general anaesthetics:

(a) initially depress higher cortical functions without causing loss of consciousness

(b) may cause impairment of cardiovascular control

(c) abolish all reflexes before the first plane of surgical anaesthesia is reached

(d) induce skeletal muscle relaxation

(e) regularly abolish respiration during the stage of surgical anaesthesia

A246 (a) **F**   The glucose-sensitive cells (in the satiety centre) are not   **6.28**
stimulated merely by the *level* of blood glucose but rather
by glucose utilization and intracellular glucose levels.
Thus diabetic patients are often constantly hungry
despite elevated blood glucose

    (b) **T**   Osmoreceptors located in the hypothalamus elicit a   **6.28**
drinking response when extracellular osmolality rises

    (c) **T**   This is recorded best over the occipital area of the cortex   **6.21**
with the eyes closed

    (d) **F**   During REM sleep the reticular formation is depressed   **6.25**
and hence there is a loss of muscle tone

    (e) **T**   This is a slow wave with a large amplitude. It is seen in   **6.22**
deep sleep and anaesthesia, and may be recorded also in
normal, waking children

A247 (a) **T**   So-called Stage 1 or the stage of analgesia; the patient   **7.2**
may experience perceptual disturbances; reflexes are
present

    (b) **T**   During Stage 2, anaesthetics with a slow rate of induc-   **7.2**
tion may have profound effects on autonomic nervous
activity (e.g. vagal inhibition; sympathetic stimulation)
and hence influence cardiovascular function

    (c) **F**   Reflexes are not totally abolished until the fourth plane   **7.2**
of surgical anaesthesia is reached

    (d) **T**   In the third plane of surgical anaesthesia the peritoneal   **7.2**
reflex is abolished and abdominal operations may be
carried out without muscle relaxants, but this is not
normal procedure

    (e) **F**   Although there may be irregularities of respiration,   **7.2**
particularly in the fourth plane of Stage 3, abolition of
respiration is not usually seen

Q248 Anaesthetic drugs:

(a) may preferentially depress the ascending reticular activating system
(b) are all highly water soluble
(c) impair neuronal function mainly by altering the nerve membrane resting potential
(d) are slowly sequestered in body fat stores
(e) given by inhalation are always used to maintain rather than induce anaesthesia

Q249 Anaesthetic agents:

(a) have structures that indicate their effect is due to interaction with specific receptors
(b) tend to be lipophilic
(c) may inhibit conduction along nerve fibres
(d) may inhibit synaptic transmission
(e) tend to be highly reactive chemically

A248 (a) **T** Although several anaesthetic drugs may depress the reticular activating system, in appropriate doses they also depress other brain regions. Regional differences in susceptibility to anaesthetics are probably due to density of blood supply, tissue lipid content and the sensitivity of the neurones to local metabolic disturbances — 7.2, 7.3

(b) **F** The common property of the anaesthetics is that they are lipid soluble — 7.3

(c) **F** Although the precise mechanisms of action are not clear, anaesthetics seem to act by impairing synaptic transmission — probably by a combination of reduced transmitter release and depressed excitability of the postsynaptic membrane — 7.5

(d) **T** Although these drugs are lipid soluble, body fat has a poor blood supply hence the concentration of drug in such sites is slow to equilibrate with the concentration in blood — 7.6

(e) **F** Although, generally, induction is achieved with an intravenous anaesthetic, the inhalation anaesthetics nitrous oxide, ethylene and cyclopropane cause rapid and pleasant induction — 7.7, 7.12

A249 (a) **F** Drugs which act as general anaesthetics show marked variation in structure, indicating their effects are non-specific — 7.3

(b) **T** Solubility in lipids is a common property of such drugs, and it may be that anaesthesia results from an interaction of the drug with cell membrane lipids — 7.3

(c) **T** Generally this occurs only with high concentrations, and is not associated with a change in membrane potential — possibly indicating an effect on Na^+ conductance — 7.5

(d) **T** This effect is particularly clear in the periphery; it is seen with relatively low concentrations and indicates that this may be the main mode of action in the nervous system — 7.5

(e) **F** Many (e.g. nitrogen, xenon) are chemically unreactive or are unable to form ionic, dipole or hydrogen bonds — 7.3

Q250 Concerning the inhalation anaesthetics:

(a)   ether causes rapid induction

(b)   chloroform tends to cause a fall in systemic arterial blood pressure

(c)   halothane tends to cause hypertension

(d)   cyclopropane causes neuromuscular blockade

(e)   in general, one of their major drawbacks is the formation of toxic decomposition products

Q251 During anaesthesia:

(a)   atropine may be given to reduce bronchial secretion

(b)   motor functions of the spinal cord are lost before sensory functions

(c)   muscle relaxants are always required in addition to the anaesthetic agent before major surgery

(d)   generalized muscular rigidity may occur in patients susceptible to malignant hyperpyrexia

(e)   ganglion-blocking drugs may be given to produce a 'bloodless field' for surgery

A250 (a) **F** Induction is very slow with ether because it is hydro- 7.9
philic and thus saturation of the blood is slow (since it
distributes rapidly in total body water)

(b) **T** Due to myocardial depression (reduced cardiac output), 7.8
inhibition of the vasomotor centre and direct peripheral
vasodilatation

(c) **F** Halothane may cause hypotension and bradycardia due 7.8
to depression of the heart, vasomotor centre and peripheral ganglionic transmission

(d) **F** In non-toxic doses, cyclopropane (and indeed, many 7.9
inhalation anaesthetics) do not produce adequate neuromuscular blockade for major surgery

(e) **T** The volatile liquid anaesthetics are readily oxidized 7.7
giving rise, for example, to phosgene and peroxides
unless stored under the right conditions

A251 (a) **T** It is also thought that atropine (or hyoscine) may protect 7.15
the heart from vagal inhibition, but the dose given is
usually too low to exert this effect

(b) **F** The opposite is true; it is not until stage 3 that the 7.2
muscles relax. In stage 2 sensory function is impaired
and there is some increased muscle tone and
exaggerated reflexes

(c) **T** Although a few anaesthetics *can* produce adequate 7.10
muscle relaxation, this is not achieved until the depth of
anaesthesia is beyond the required level

(d) **T** In addition to the rise in body temperature, metabolic 7.11
acidosis and muscular rigidity occur; this has been attributed to an impairment in Ca^{2+} binding to the sarcoplasmic reticulum such that the anaesthetic promotes
excessive Ca^{2+} release

(e) **T** The rapid onset, short-acting drugs (trimetaphan) are 7.15,
used for this purpose 10.24

Q252 Considering the intravenous anaesthetics:

(a) the short-acting barbiturate sodium thiopentone causes rapid induction because of its low lipid-water solubility coefficient

(b) the short-acting barbiturates tend to cause respiratory depression

(c) ketamine may cause marked psychic effects in adults

(d) the steroid preparation althesin is rapidly metabolized by the liver

(e) propanidid has a short duration of action because it is rapidly metabolized by the kidney

Q253 Considering hypnotics and sedatives:

(a) the hypnotic chloral hydrate blocks neuromuscular transmission when taken orally

(b) the hypnotic paraldehyde is routinely administered intravenously

(c) the hypnotic glutethimide may produce dependence after chronic administration

(d) the benzodiazepines are of particular value in insomnia due to anxiety

(e) the barbiturates may cause disturbance of sleep pattern

A252 (a) **F** Sodium thiopentone has an exceptionally high lipid-   **7.12**
water solubility coefficient and hence is rapidly taken up
by the brain

(b) **T** These drugs (e.g. thiopentone, methohexitone, hexo-   **7.12**
barbitone) may cause depression of the respiratory
centre, and the means of treating these problems should
always be at hand

(c) **T** Vivid dreams, delirium, confusion and irrational   **7.13**
behaviour occur in many adult patients (c.f. effects of
phencyclidine); these effects are less marked or absent
in children

(d) **T** The drug is metabolized by the enzyme systems respon-   **7.14**
sible for handling endogenous steroids

(e) **F** Propanidid is rapidly metabolized by plasma and liver   **7.13**
esterases (into a derivative of phenylacetic acid and
propanol)

A253 (a) **F** Although chloral hydrate is a potent anticholinesterase   **8.2**
and can *antagonize* the actions of tubocurarine, its
active metabolite trichloroethanol has no such effects

(b) **F** Paraldehyde may be administered orally, intramus-   **8.3**
cularly or rectally; paraldehyde dissolves plastics and
disposable plastic syringes should not be used for its
administration.

(c) **T** A property in common with those of other hypnotics and   **8.10**
sedatives; usual withdrawal symptoms include nausea,
vomiting, weakness, hypotension, anxiety, etc.

(d) **T** Reverberating neuronal activity of the limbic system   **8.11**
(associated with anxiety) can activate the brain stem
reticular system and maintain wakefulness; benzodiazepines suppress this effect

(e) **T** Barbiturates initially depress the proportion of REM   **8.7**
sleep; when withdrawn there may be REM rebound

Q254 Barbiturate drugs:

    (a)   produce their sedative effect by directly depressing synaptic transmission

    (b)   have a quicker onset and shorter duration of action the more lipid soluble they are

    (c)   are useful analgesics

    (d)   given in anaesthetic doses increase urine flow

    (e)   are excreted more rapidly in an alkaline urine

Q255 Drugs in the barbiturate group:

    (a)   may be used as anticonvulsants

    (b)   may be used as hypnotics or sedatives

    (c)   may be used as anaesthetics

    (d)   have analgesic properties

    (e)   when taken repeatedly may induce tolerance to their actions

A254 (a) **T** This probably arises from a combination of reduced transmitter release and depressed postsynaptic membrane sensitivity 8.5

(b) **T** There are three main groups of barbiturates described on the basis of duration of action. Those in group 3 are the most lipid soluble hence quickly penetrate to their site of action in the brain 8.7

(c) **F** Unless given in anaesthetic doses, the barbiturates do not prevent the sense of pain — indeed in small doses they may produce hyperalgesia 8.7

(d) **F** They reduce urine flow — probably due to a combination of reduced filtration (secondary to hypotension) and stimulation of the release of antidiuretic hormone 8.8

(e) **T** The pKa is between 7 and 8; thus an increase in pH increases the fraction of drug in the ionized form (more water soluble) and reduces the rate of reabsorption from the tubules — this may be taken advantage of in cases of barbiturate poisoning 8.9

A255 (a) **T** Those compounds with slow onset and long duration of action (e.g.phenobarbitone) have a selective anticonvulsant effect in doses which produce minimal sedation 8.7

(b) **T** Those with an intermediate duration of action are used as sedatives and, in doses 3–4 times greater, as hypnotics 8.7

(c) **T** The short-acting, rapid onset barbiturates (e.g. methohexitone) are used as intravenous anaesthetics 8.7

(d) **F** In small doses they may cause hyperalgesia. In the presence of pain they do not produce sedation or sleep — instead they may cause restlessness 8.8

(e) **T** This is due to a lesser central nervous effect at the same blood level (pharmacodynamic tolerance) and to enzyme induction leading to more rapid metabolism 8.8

Q256 Benzodiazepines:

(a)   exert their sedative effect principally by acting on the reticular activating system
(b)   can act centrally as muscle relaxants
(c)   may be used in the treatment of alcohol and other drug withdrawal syndromes
(d)   increase the proportion of REM sleep
(e)   may be used as anti-epileptics

Q257 Benzodiazepines:

(a)   may cause an increase in skeletal muscle tone
(b)   may be useful in myoclonic epilepsy
(c)   do not disturb the proportion of non-REM to REM sleep
(d)   caused marked antagonism of monoamine transmission in the central nervous system
(e)   have useful anti-anxiety effects

A256 (a) **F** Their main site of action is on the limbic system — they appear to suppress the ability of the limbic system to activate the reticular formation   **8.11**

(b) **T** This can occur at the supraspinal and spinal level and may involve stimulation of glycine receptors (glycine functions as an inhibitory transmitter in the CNS)   **18.16**

(c) **T** The sedative effects of benzodiazepines serve to lessen the intensity of the symptoms of withdrawal (mainly signs of excessive sympathetic activity)   **42.16, 42.17**

(d) **F** The benzodiazepines affect sleep patterns to a lesser extent than barbiturates, but any effect is a reduction in REM sleep   **8.11**

(e) **T** The mechanism of action is not well understood, but part of their anti-epileptic action may be attributable to their ability to stimulate inhibitory glycine receptors   **8.11, 18.28, 18.32**

A257 (a) **F** Benzodiazepine tranquillizers (e.g. diazepam and lorazepam) depress spinal reflexes and also suppress supraspinal input to skeletal muscle, thereby reducing tone   **18.16**

(b) **T** Myoclonic epilepsy (characterized by brief, jerky movements, without loss of consciousness) is susceptible to large doses of diazepam or clonazepam (see (a))   **18.26**

(c) **F** Benzodiazepines such as nitrazepam and flurazepam do influence the balance of REM to non-REM sleep (as do barbiturates). However, this effect is much less marked than with other hypnotics   **8.11**

(d) **F** Benzodiazepines are largely devoid of effects on central neurotransmission involving monoamines or acetylcholine. Consistent with this, they have little effect on autonomic neurotransmission in the periphery   **15.21**

(e) **T** These drugs appear to cause a relatively specific depression of activity in the limbic system. This results in reduced emotional reactivity and the associated restlessness, tremor and palpitations   **15.21**

Central Nervous System   233

Q258 Ethanol:

  (a) taken in small quantities (to give blood levels of about 10 mM) is a central nervous system stimulant
  (b) stimulates gastric secretion
  (c) stimulates the secretion of antidiuretic hormone
  (d) increases core temperature
  (e) absorption from the gastrointestinal tract is delayed by the presence of food in the stomach

Q259 Ethanol:

  (a) tends to cause vasoconstriction
  (b) inhibits gastric acid secretion when ingested in low (<10%) concentrations
  (c) causes diuresis due to inhibition of antidiuretic hormone secretion
  (d) is initially metabolized to acetaldehyde, mainly in the liver
  (e) may induce tolerance to barbiturates

Q260 In the central nervous system:

  (a) most of the acetylcholine (ACh) in the spinal cord is located in the anterior roots and horns
  (b) acetylcholine in the brain acts only on nicotinic receptors
  (c) the biosynthesis of serotonin depends on the plasma level of tyrosine
  (d) the distribution of dopamine closely parallels that of noradrenaline
  (e) a large proportion of the noradrenaline is of peripheral origin

A258 (a) **F** Ethanol is entirely depressant; the apparent 'stimulant' 8.12
effects are due to depression of the integrating activity of
the reticular formation which frees the cortex from some
inhibitory control

(b) **T** This occurs through the release of histamine and gastrin 8.13
and is partly responsible for the appetite-stimulant
effect of ethanol

(c) **F** It reduces ADH secretion, thus facilitating diuresis 8.13

(d) **F** Despite a feeling of warmth due to flushed skin, a periph- 8.13
eral vasodilatation increases heat loss; furthermore,
large doses of ethanol may depress hypothalamic
temperature-regulating mechanisms, making the fall in
temperature more severe

(e) **T** Ethanol is rapidly absorbed from the fasted stomach, 8.13
intestine and colon; milk is (believed to be) particularly
effective in delaying absorption

A259 (a) **F** Ethanol causes vasodilatation under normal conditions, 8.13
due to inhibition of the vasomotor centre

(b) **F** Alcohol ingestion normally stimulates gastric acid secre- 8.13
tion, due to release of histamine and gastrin

(c) **T** Ethanol-induced inhibition of antidiuretic hormone 8.13
secretion prevents the excretion of a concentrated urine

(d) **T** The enzyme alcohol dehydrogenase is responsible for 8.13
this conversion

(e) **T** This is partly due to adaptive changes in the central 8.14
nervous system but also because ethanol increases
hepatic microsomal enzyme activity responsible for
barbiturate metabolism

A260 (a) **T** These regions contain the highest ACh content of any 14.8
area in the CNS consistent with the location of
cholinergic axons and cell bodies of cholinergic motoneurones in these regions

(b) **F** Both muscarinic and nicotinic receptors are found in the 14.5
CNS; activation of these receptors may have excitatory
or inhibitory effects

(c) **F** Dopamine and noradrenaline biosynthesis in the CNS 14.8
starts with the uptake of tyrosine; serotonin biosynthesis
depends on the uptake of tryptophan

(d) **F** There are several regions where dopamine-β-hydroxy- 14.10
lase activity is low and the concentration of dopamine is
far higher than that of noradrenaline; in such areas
dopamine may function as a neurotransmitter in its own
right

(e) **F** The blood–brain barrier is impermeable to cate- 14.8
cholamines and serotonin

Q261 Neuroleptic phenothiazines:

    (a)   are effective in the treatment of nausea and vomiting, whatever the cause

    (b)   may exert an antipsychotic effect in schizophrenia

    (c)   are effective in the treatment of psychotic reactions induced by atropine-like drugs

    (d)   are often useful in the treatment of anxiety neuroses

    (e)   when ingested, are preferentially accumulated in the cerebral cortex

Q262 In man, chlorpromazine:

    (a)   produces a sedative effect due to its preferential accumulation in the cerebral cortex

    (b)   potentiates the depressant effects of anaesthetics

    (c)   is an effective treatment for motion sickness

    (d)   often predisposes to postural hypotension and tachycardia

    (e)   may increase prolactin secretion by inhibiting the action of dopamine

A261 (a) **F** Chlorpromazine depresses the medullary chemo- **15.9**
receptor trigger zone and suppresses vomiting due to
apomorphine, ergot alkaloids, pregnancy and labyrin-
thine disease. It is ineffective against vomiting provoked
by cardiac glycosides, copper sulphate, X-irradiation or
motion

     (b) **T** These drugs markedly reduce the frequency, duration **15.8**
and severity of schizophrenic episodes. Furthermore
they tend to abolish the usual manifestations of the
disorder (abnormal thought processes, delusions,
hallucinations, withdrawal, etc.)

     (c) **F** Although these drugs are useful in the psychotic reac- **15.9**
tions induced by amphetamine, lysergide and related
compounds, they may exacerbate the central nervous
effects of atropine-like drugs (e.g. scopolamine)

     (d) **T** For this purpose, the drugs are used in smaller doses **15.9**
than are needed to exert an antipsychotic effect. They
reduce the tension, excitation or aggression that may be
associated with anxiety states

     (e) **F** These drugs tend to be accumulated in those parts of the **15.6**
brain associated with alertness and performance (limbic
system, hypothalamus, thalamus)

A262 (a) **F** Chlorpromazine does exert a sedative effect, but this is **15.6**
by way of preferentially accumulating in areas con-
cerned with alertness and performance, i.e. reticular-
activating system, limbic system, hypothalamus and
thalamus

     (b) **T** Although large doses of chlorpromazine do not have an **15.6**
anaesthetic effect, they do potentiate the effects of
anaesthetics, hypnotics and sedatives

     (c) **F** Although it does have antiemetic effects by depressing **15.9,**
the chemoreceptor trigger zone of the medulla, it does **25.7**
not suppress vomiting due to motion sickness

     (d) **T** Since the drug has peripheral α-adrenoceptor anta- **15.10**
gonist properties, as well as atropine-like effects, this
combination is probably responsible for the cardiovascular effects

     (e) **T** Chlorpromazine is a relatively potent dopamine anta- **15.11,**
gonist; it therefore blocks the inhibitory effect of dopa- **15.5**
mine on prolactin secretion. As a result gynaecomastia
(in men) and galactorrhoea (in women) may occur

Q263 Drugs in the phenothiazine group:

(a) may induce an anaesthetic state when given in large doses

(b) are used to control vomiting due to vestibular dysfunction

(c) may cause postural hypotension

(d) may produce diarrhoea

(e) may produce blurred vision

Q264 Drugs in the phenothiazine group:

(a) may produce hypothermia

(b) may inhibit skeletal neuromuscular transmission

(c) may produce increased prolactin levels in the plasma

(d) may produce jaundice

(e) may lead to skin pigmentation

A263 (a) **F** The phenothiazines are major 'tranquillizers' which may have a sedative effect, but arousal can be produced by moderate stimulation (unlike sedative-hypnotics)   **15.6**

(b) **T** They depress the chemoreceptor trigger zone of the medulla and are effective against vomiting due to Ménière's disease   **15.9**

(c) **T** These effects are largely due to α-adrenoceptor antagonism, and inhibition of hypothalamic cardiovascular control mechanisms   **15.10**

(d) **F** Constipation may occur due to an atropine-like effect on the gut. Such effects may be exacerbated when other atropine-like drugs are given to alleviate the extra-pyramidal side-effects of phenothiazines   **15.10**

(e) **T** Atropine-like effects on parasympathetic control of the iris and ciliary muscles are probably responsible   **15.10**

A264 (a) **T** Impairment of hypothalamic mechanisms and loss of peripheral vasoconstrictor tone (due to α-adrenoceptor antagonism) leads to a fall in body temperature under normal ambient conditions   **15.10**

(b) **F** Disorders of motor control seen with phenothiazines (extrapyramidal effects) are likely to be due to interference with dopaminergic transmission from nerve terminals of cell bodies in the substantia nigra (c.f. Parkinsonism)   **15.10**

(c) **T** The dopaminergic inhibition of prolactin release from the pituitary is suppressed by phenothiazines; this leads to swelling of the breasts in males and lactation in females   **15.11**

(d) **T** Obstructive jaundice may be produced by chlorpromazine (incidence of 1 in about 200) but is uncommon with other phenothiazines   **15.11, 26.33–26.34**

(e) **T** Increased melanin deposition (due to increased release of melanocyte-stimulating hormone) and deposition of phenothiazine metabolites are responsible   **15.11**

Q265 Tricyclic antidepressants:

    (a)   are more potent than the neuroleptic phenothiazines at blocking prejunctional uptake of noradrenaline and serotonin

    (b)   are less potent than the neuroleptic phenothiazines at blocking postjunctional receptors

    (c)   exhibit a rapid onset of action

    (d)   potentiate the antihypertensive effect of guanethidine

    (e)   may cause blurred vision

Q266 The tricyclic antidepressant group of drugs:

    (a)   inhibit the neuronal uptake of noradrenaline

    (b)   have a rapid onset of action

    (c)   may cause constipation and dry mouth

    (d)   do not produce postural hypotension

    (e)   may produce tachycardia and palpitations

A265 (a) **T** Block of prejunctional uptake of noradrenaline and serotonin probably makes more available to act on postjunctional receptors   **15.15**

(b) **T** The relative lack of antagonism of postjunctional receptors together with the blockade of prejunctional uptake probably acts to enhance noradrenergic and serotoninergic transmission. Phenothiazines act predominantly by blocking postjunctional receptors   **15.15**

(c) **F** The characteristic feature of these drugs is that they are slow in onset, taking up to two weeks of continual treatment before benefit accrues; the reason for this is unclear   **15.17**

(d) **F** They antagonize this effect — probably because the adrenergic neurone blocking activity of drugs such as guanethidine depends on sequestration in the nerve terminals, and this uptake process would be blocked by the tricyclic antidepressants   **15.18**

(e) **T** These drugs have atropine-like actions which are responsible for their side-effects on vision   **15.17, 29.13**

A266 (a) **T** This effect is generally much more marked than is seen with the phenothiazines; it is not clear if this action is responsible for the antidepressant effect   **15.16**

(b) **F** Their antidepressant action is slow in onset (up to two weeks after initiation of treatment) — the reasons for this are unclear   **15.17**

(c) **T** These are probably due to the atropine-like effects of the drugs   **15.17**

(d) **F** Postural hypotension is not uncommon with these drugs and may be due to α-adrenoceptor antagonism and effects on medullary vasomotor reflex mechanisms   **15.17**

(e) **T** Probably due to enhanced sympathetic drive (due to inhibition of noradrenaline uptake) and inhibition of vagal tone (an atropine-like effect)   **15.17**

Q267 Monoamine oxidase inhibitors:

(a) inhibit the action of several drugs
(b) may predispose to postural hypotension
(c) produce blurred vision due to a potent atropine-like action
(d) may cause hypertension in patients taking amphetamines
(e) may cause hepatotoxicity

Q268 Monoamine oxidase (MAO) inhibitors:

(a) are routinely used in the treatment of endogenous depression
(b) tend to cause hypertension
(c) may cause dry mouth, constipation and blurring of vision
(d) of the hydrazine group may produce hepatotoxicity
(e) show little interaction with other drugs

A267 (a) **F** These drugs inhibit a number of enzymes in addition to monoamine oxidase. Their effect in inhibiting microsomal enzyme activity results in potentiation of the action of a number of drugs which depend on microsomal enzymes for terminating their action. In some cases this is beneficial whereas in others it is detrimental **15.19, 26.21– 26.22**

(b) **T** Postural hypotension is a common side-effect of these drugs — indeed some are used in the treatment of hypertension although their mechanism of action is unclear **15.19, 23.49– 23.50**

(c) **F** Blurred vision is a side-effect of these drugs but they have little or no atropine-like activity. The visual impairment is probably due to a diminution of central parasympathetic drive **15.19**

(d) **T** These drugs do not greatly affect responses to exogenous noradrenaline (which is removed principally by neuronal uptake), but they do greatly potentiate the effects of indirectly acting sympathomimetics **11.10, 11.11**

(e) **T** Jaundice is a side-effect of these drugs, and for this reason iproniazid was withdrawn from the US market, although the incidence of fatal hepatotoxicity is very low **15.19, 26.36**

A268 (a) **F** MAO inhibitors do not work well in endogenous depression, but are often effective in reactive depression (e.g. following bereavement) **15.10**

(b) **F** Although they inhibit the metabolism of monoamines they do not augment peripheral vasoconstrictor tone (the reasons for this are debatable (**23.49–50**)), but cause postural hypotension **15.19**

(c) **T** Although these effects are atropine-like, MAO inhibitors have little such activity; it is possible the effects are due to central inhibition of parasympathetic tone **15.19**

(d) **T** The incidence of side-effect is low, but mortality is high; it is likely that the hepatic damage is due to reactive metabolites (**26.36**) **15.19**

(e) **F** Interactions between MAO inhibitors and other drugs are extensive; furthermore they may produce problems with substances ingested in food **15.19**

Q269 The analgesic drug morphine may cause:

(a) nausea and vomiting
(b) hypotension
(c) dilatation of the pupils
(d) polyuria
(e) bronchoconstriction

Q270 In man, morphine:

(a) inhibits the release of antidiuretic hormone
(b) may cause difficulty with urination
(c) may cause vomiting
(d) increases gastrointestinal motility
(e) is readily absorbed following oral ingestion

Q271 In man, morphine:

(a) readily crosses the blood–brain barrier
(b) reduces the sensitivity of peripheral pain receptors
(c) may be used in the treatment of diarrhoea
(d) reduces the sensitivity of the brain stem respiratory centres to hypoxia
(e) exerts a direct antitussive action

A269 (a) **T** Morphine initially stimulates the chemoreceptor trigger zone in the medulla causing nausea and vomiting; it subsequently depresses the vomiting centre   16.3

(b) **T** Due to depression of the vasomotor centre and stimulation of the vagal efferent outflow   16.3

(c) **F** Morphine causes miosis partly due to enhancement of the pupillary light reflex, but also to stimulation of neurones in the Edinger-Westphal nucleus   16.3

(d) **F** Morphine stimulates antidiuretic hormone release and hence reduces the rate of formation of urine; it also causes detrusor and vesicle sphincter contraction causing urinary urgency and difficulty in urination   16.3

(e) **T** Partly due to histamine release; this may be troublesome in respiratory insufficiency (asthma and emphysema)   16.3

A270 (a) **F** Morphine produces an antidiuretic effect by stimulating the release of ADH from the posterior pituitary   16.3, 27.39

(b) **T** It increases the tone of the detrusor muscle causing 'urinary urgency', but increases the tone of the sphincter causing difficulty with urination   16.3

(c) **T** Morphine can cause nausea and vomiting through stimulation of the chemoreceptor trigger zone — this may then be followed by inhibition of vomiting due to an action of morphine on the vomiting centre   16.3

(d) **F** It reduces motility and increases tone in the gastrointestinal tract, with contraction of the sphincters leading to constipation   16.3

(e) **F** It is poorly absorbed after oral ingestion and for this reason is usually given subcutaneously, intramuscularly or intravenously   16.3

A271 (a) **F** Although the brain is the main site of action of morphine, relatively little of an administered dose penetrates the blood–brain barrier   16.3

(b) **F** Morphine does not affect sensory receptor sensitivity or afferent fibre signalling; it probably exerts its analgesic action at the level of the spinal cord and/or brain   16.4

(c) **T** Propulsive peristalsis through the gastrointestinal tract is reduced allowing more time for water reabsorption   16.4

(d) **F** The medullary respiratory centre is sensitive to $[H^+]$ which is elevated by an increase in P_{CO_2}. Morphine depresses this sensitivity with the result that the main stimulus to breathing becomes hypoxia   16.4, 24.10

(e) **T** Morphine directly depresses the cough centre in the medulla through an action unrelated to its analgesic or respiratory depressant action   16.5, 24.10

Q272   The analgesic drug morphine:

(a)   is readily absorbed after oral ingestion
(b)   has no effect on the sensitivity of pain receptors
(c)   increases peristalsis in the small intestine
(d)   in normal therapeutic doses depresses respiration
(e)   induces tolerance with repeated dosing

Q273   In man:

(a)   diamorphine has a less potent antitussive effect than morphine
(b)   diamorphine is more readily absorbed than morphine after oral ingestion
(c)   codeine taken in large doses produces central nervous depression
(d)   codeine is rapidly metabolized after oral ingestion
(e)   apomorphine may be used as an emetic

Q274   The analgesic drug:

(a)   diamorphine is better absorbed than morphine after oral ingestion
(b)   codeine possesses antitussive and antidiarrhoeal actions
(c)   etorphine is less potent than morphine in reducing pain
(d)   pethidine has a longer duration of action than morphine
(e)   methadone does not produce tolerance and dependence with repeated use

A272 (a) **F** Morphine is not well absorbed from the gastrointestinal   **16.3**
tract; it is usually given by subcutaneous, intramuscular
or intravenous injection

(b) **T** The site of analgesic action may be in the spinal cord   **16.4**
and/or brain, but an effect on receptors or afferent fibre
signalling is absent

(c) **F** Morphine increases the tone of the antral portion of the   **16.4**
stomach and of the small and large intestines, but
propulsive peristalsis is decreased

(d) **T** This effect is due to a decrease in the sensitivity of   **16.4**
medullary chemoreceptors to CO_2 and H^+; under these
conditions hypoxia stimulates ventilation

(e) **T** This is characterized by decreased intensity and   **16.5**
duration of effects and elevation of the lethal dose

A273 (a) **F** The opposite is true, and in some countries diamorphine   **16.6**
is still used as a cough suppressant

(b) **T** This is because it is more lipid soluble. Once absorbed it   **16.6**
is converted to morphine and it is likely that most of its
pharmacological actions are due to the morphine
generated

(c) **F** Unlike morphine, large doses of codeine produce excita-   **16.7**
tion of central nervous structures

(d) **F** Codeine is only slowly metabolized and this contributes   **16.7**
to its relatively greater oral efficacy compared to
morphine. About 10% of the codeine is metabolized to
morphine

(e) **T** Apomorphine is a less potent analgesic than morphine   **16.9**
but it still possesses the capacity to stimulate the
medullary chemoreceptor trigger zone giving rise to
vomiting

A274 (a) **T** It is more lipid-soluble than morphine; it is converted into   **16.6**
morphine after absorption

(b) **T** As does morphine; however, it has less analgesic effect   **16.7**
than morphine and rarely produces serious dependence

(c) **F** In man the analgesic effect of etorphine is about 200   **16.8**
times that of morphine; it produces less respiratory
depression, nausea and vomiting

(d) **F** Pethidine is less potent and has a shorter duration of   **16.9**
action than morphine; the usual dose (50–100 mg) has
effects that last 2–4 h

(e) **F** Methadone produces tolerance and dependence of the   **16.9**
morphine type, thus morphine addicts do not show withdrawal symptoms if given methadone

Q275 Compared to morphine, pethidine:

    (a)   has a shorter duration of action

    (b)   produces a similar degree of pupillary constriction

    (c)   is less likely to induce tolerance and dependence

    (d)   is more likely to give rise to hallucinations and convulsions

    (e)   is more likely to cause dry mouth and thirst

Q276 Compared to morphine, methadone:

    (a)   is more potent as a respiratory depressant

    (b)   is less effective when taken by mouth

    (c)   does not give rise to tolerance and dependence with prolonged use

    (d)   gives rise to similar withdrawal symptoms on cessation of use

    (e)   has a more powerful sedative effect

Q277 In man, pentazocine:

    (a)   is equipotent to morphine in its analgesic action

    (b)   produces a similar degree of hypotension and bradycardia as morphine

    (c)   causes less severe respiratory depression than morphine

    (d)   precipitates the withdrawal syndrome when given following prolonged morphine treatment

    (e)   overdosage is most effectively treated with naloxone

A275 (a) **T** The effects of an average dose (50–100 mg) last for about 2 to 4 h; this is advantageous when used in labour since respiratory depression in the neonate will be less prolonged   **16.9**

(b) **F** This effect is less because pethidine also has atropine-like effects   **16.9**

(c) **F** Pethidine is equivalent to morphine in this respect, giving rise to morphine-type symptoms of tolerance and dependence   **16.9**

(d) **T** Norpethidine is one of the metabolites of pethidine and is thought to be responsible for the excitatory effects on the central nervous system   **16.9**

(e) **T** This is another manifestion of the atropine-like effects of this drug (see (b))   **16.9**

A276 (a) **T** It is a slightly more potent analgesic but is considerably more potent in its effect on respiration and coughing   **16.9**

(b) **F** Unlike morphine, methadone is almost as active by mouth as by parenteral administration   **16.9**

(c) **F** With prolonged use, tolerance and dependence of the morphine type develop   **16.9**

(d) **F** Because methadone has a longer duration of action, the methadone withdrawal syndrome is slower in onset (and longer in duration) but much less intense. Hence methadone can be used in the treatment of morphine dependence since the two drugs show cross tolerance and methadone can be substituted for morphine without precipitating morphine withdrawal symptoms   **16.10**

(e) **F** The sedative action of methadone is slightly weaker than that of morphine   **16.9**

A277 (a) **F** It is 3–4 times less potent than morphine as an analgesic. It also possesses antagonist activity but in this respect it is about 50 times less potent than nalorphine   **16.13**

(b) **F** Unlike morphine, pentazocine causes hypertension (systemic and pulmonary) and tachycardia. This is possibly due to the fact that it increases plasma catecholamine levels   **16.14, Table 16.1**

(c) **T** However, with very high doses respiration is depressed. This effect is antagonized by naloxone but not by nalorphine   **16.14**

(d) **T** This is because of its antagonist activity, although it is much weaker than nalorphine in this respect   **16.13**

(e) **T** Naloxone is a pure antagonist and is useful in acute morphine poisoning and overdosage with similar drugs   **16.13, 16.14**

Q278 The drug:

(a) nalorphine acts as a partial agonist at opiate receptors

(b) pentazocine is more effective than morphine in relieving severe pain

(c) naloxone may be used in the treatment of acute morphine poisoning

(d) naltrexone is a less potent opiate antagonist than naloxone

(e) pentazocine, like morphine, produces constipation

Q279 Drugs in the 'salicylate' group are:

(a) rapidly absorbed from the stomach

(b) only slowly absorbed from the alkaline contents of the small intestine

(c) more rapidly excreted in an acid urine than in an alkaline urine

(d) metabolized chiefly in the liver

(e) secreted into tubular fluid by proximal tubular cells

A278 (a) **T** It has an antagonist effect when administered in the presence of a morphine-like analgesic but is about equipotent with morphine as an analgesic   **16.12**

(b) **F** It is 3–4 times less potent than morphine as an analgesic, but its antagonistic effects give it advantages over morphine in situations where the production of dependence is particularly undesirable   **16.13**

(c) **T** Naloxone is a pure morphine antagonist and is very effective in reversing the effects of morphine overdosage, e.g. respiratory depression   **16.14**

(d) **F** Naltrexone is about 8 times as potent as naloxone, and is also active orally   **16.14**

(e) **F** The constipation and biliary spasm frequently seen with morphine are rarely observed with pentazocine   **16.14**

A279 (a) **T** The pKa of salicylates is low and therefore they are mainly in the non-ionized, more lipid-soluble form at the low pH in the stomach   **16.19**

(b) **F** Although the salicylates are predominantly ionized in this alkaline environment, the surface area (for absorption) is so great the rate of absorption exceeds that in the stomach   **16.19**

(c) **F** In alkaline urine about 85% of the administered dose is excreted as unchanged salicylate whereas in acid urine ionization is suppressed and the non-ionized lipid-soluble form is partly reabsorbed   **16.20**

(d) **T** The main metabolic products are gentisic acid (up to 5%), salicyluric acid (up to 50%), o-hydroxybenzoyl glucuronide ether (up to 10%) and o-carboxyphenolglucuronide ether (10–30%)   **16.20**

(e) **T** This process is dependent upon a carrier-facilitated transport mechanism handling weak organic acids   **16.20**

Q280 In man, salicylates:

(a) are more potent analgesics in conditions where plasma protein levels are low

(b) are excreted more rapidly in an alkaline urine

(c) do not cross the placenta

(d) may stimulate respiration

(e) may increase plasma bicarbonate concentration

Q281 Acetylsalicylic acid (aspirin):

(a) exerts an analgesic action and antipyretic effect at a similar dose

(b) may cause sedation through its action on the reticular activating system

(c) inhibits prostaglandin synthesis

(d) increases platelet adhesiveness

(e) may lead to iron-deficiency anaemia after prolonged use

A280 (a) **T** 50–80% of salicylic acid in plasma is protein bound, and   **16.20**
only the free form is active. Thus when plasma protein
(especially albumin) is low, such as in rheumatoid
arthritis or in children, there is more drug in the free
state and more is concentrated in tissues

(b) **T** If distal tubular urine is acid, ionization of salicylic acid   **16.20**
is suppressed and the non-ionized lipid-soluble form is
partly reabsorbed. In alkaline urine most of the salicylic
acid is ionized and the salicylate ion is retained in the
urine

(c) **F** Salicylate penetrates into CSF, synovial fluid, peritoneal   **16.19**
fluid, saliva and milk and readily crosses the placental
barrier

(d) **T** This is due to a combination of increased CO_2 production   **16.23**
(due to increased cellular metabolism) and a direct
effect of salicylates on the respiratory centre. It is a
clear characteristic of salicylate poisoning

(e) **F** The hyperventilation [see(d)] results in respiratory   **16.23**
alkalosis which is partly compensated by the kidneys
leading to a reduction in plasma bicarbonate. In this
compensated situation the patient is then more susceptible to the toxic effects of higher doses of salicylates
since the body's buffering capacity has been reduced

A281 (a) **T** The analgesic dose (0.3–1 g every 3–4 h) is lower than   **16.21**
the anti-inflammatory dose

(b) **F** The analgesic effect is not associated with changes in   **16.21**
mood or arousal. Because of the paucity of central
nervous effects it has been suggested that the main site
of analgesic action is peripheral

(c) **T** This action may account for the antipyretic, analgesic   **16.21**
and anti-inflammatory effects of aspirin

(d) **F** The converse is true; as a result bleeding time is   **16.22,**
increased. Aspirin also lowers plasma free fatty acid   **21.22**
and cholesterol concentrations so it is potentially useful
in prophylactic treatment of ischaemic heart disease
and stroke

(e) **T** Gastric bleeding is a common side-effect seen with con-   **16.22**
tinued aspirin treatment. Ingestion of 3 g per day for 3 to
6 days results in an average blood loss of about 5 ml/day;
this blood loss may then lead to iron deficiency anaemia
if treatment with aspirin is continued

Q282 Drugs in the 'salicylate' group:

(a) may be used in the treatment of rheumatoid arthritis
(b) tend to lower normal body temperature
(c) cause analgesia by suppression of transmission through central pain pathways
(d) are prone to cause tolerance and dependence
(e) cause irritation of the gastric mucosa

Q283 The 'salicylate' group of drugs:

(a) decrease platelet adhesiveness
(b) increase plasma cortisol levels
(c) in moderate doses stimulate respiration
(d) in moderate doses lead to decreased bicarbonate excretion by the kidneys
(e) in large doses lead to metabolic acidosis

A282 (a) **T** Salicylates suppress the painful inflammatory com- **16.21**
ponent of the disease, mainly by inhibiting the
biosynthesis of prostaglandins

(b) **F** These drugs only lower abnormally raised body **16.21**
temperatures, probably by inhibition of prostaglandin
synthesis in the hypothalamus

(c) **F** Most evidence indicates that salicylates have an **16.21**
important action on peripheral pain mechanisms
(possibly by interfering with the synergy between prostaglandins and bradykinin on pain afferents)

(d) **F** Their analgesic effect against low-grade, aching pain is **16.21**
unaccompanied by narcosis, euphoria or other central
effects; tolerance and dependence are not seen

(e) **T** Discrete ulcerative and haemorrhagic lesions are **16.22**
produced, probably because high levels of the drug are
reached inside the mucosal cells

A283 (a) **T** They may also cause hypoprothrombinaemia (reversible **16.23**
with vitamin K_1); these effects may be troublesome in
some patients receiving large doses of the drug

(b) **T** Salicylates enhance ACTH release from the anterior **16.23**
pituitary and thus evoke increased cortisol release from
the adrenal cortex. However, this effect is not essential
for their anti-inflammatory actions

(c) **T** The effect is due to a direct action on the respiratory **16.23**
centre (increasing rate) and an indirect action through
increased CO_2 production (increasing depth of
respiration)

(d) **F** Respiratory stimulation leads to respiratory alkalosis **16.23**
which is compensated by renal bicarbonate excretion

(e) **T** Due to accumulation of salicylic acid, vascular collapse **16.23**
leading to renal insufficiency, and increased generation
of metabolic acids

Q284 Parkinsonism:

    (a)   may be associated with muscle rigidity

    (b)   can be induced by phenothiazines

    (c)   is associated with lesions in the motor cortex

    (d)   is associated with a reduced urinary excretion of dopamine and its metabolites

    (e)   may be induced by the antihypertensive drug α-methyldopa

Q285 In the condition known as Parkinsonism:

    (a)   there is a flaccid paralysis of skeletal muscle

    (b)   there is an involuntary tremor of resting muscles

    (c)   there may be difficulty in chewing and swallowing

    (d)   there is usually degeneration of dopaminergic neurones in the substantia nigra

    (e)   there is usually degeneration of cholinergic neurones in the striatum

A284 (a) **T** This may be due to excessive inhibitory influences leading to enhanced γ motor neurone activity and tonic stretch reflexes or it may involve excessive α motor neurone activity which is not triggered from the muscle spindles   **18.17**

(b) **T** This effect may be explained by the blocking action of these drugs at dopamine receptor sites   **18.24, 15.10**

(c) **F** The precise cause of Parkinsonism is unclear but it is associated with lesions in the basal ganglia — especially the corpus striatum   **18.18**

(d) **T** There is a deficiency in the dopamine content of the corpus striatum of Parkinsonian patients at postmortem. This, together with reduced dopamine excretion has led to the suggestion that a disturbance in dopamine activity may be the underlying cause   **18.18**

(e) **T** This drug is metabolized into a false transmitter (in the corpus striatum α-methyldopamine is formed, which then displaces dopamine from the storage granules); when released this false transmitter has a lesser effect on the receptors than dopamine itself, leading to the symptoms of dopamine deficiency   **18.24**

A285 (a) **F** Muscles are tonically contracted due to impaired central inhibitory mechanisms (possibly due to excessive γ motorneurone activity and enhanced stretch reflexes)   **18.17**

(b) **T** Mainly in the ankles and hands; in the latter it frequently involves the thumb and index finger   **18.17**

(c) **T** The disorder in these motor mechanisms may lead to nutritional deficiency   **18.18**

(d) **T** The loss of these neurones leads to denervation of the striatum to which they project   **18.18**

(e) **F** There is no detectable abnormality of cholinergic neurones; it is possible that the loss of dopaminergic elements leaves the cholinergic system unopposed, thus causing the abnormalities in muscular control   **18.18**

Q286 Some of the symptoms of Parkinsonism may be alleviated by:

(a) atropine-like drugs
(b) systemic administration of dopamine
(c) levodopa, but hypertension may ensue
(d) α-methyldopa
(e) amantidine

Q287 In the treatment of Parkinsonism:

(a) L-dopa is the drug of choice if the condition was induced by phenothiazines
(b) one aim of therapy is to reduce cholinergic activity
(c) dexamphetamine in combination with an atropine-like drug is of major benefit
(d) L-dopa often predisposes to postural hypotension
(e) L-dopa combined with an atropine-like drug is therapeutically effective

A286 (a) **T** Parasympathetic effects (salivation, sweating, incontinence) are reduced as is muscle rigidity; hypokinesia is less affected and tremor may be worsened   **18.18**

(b) **F** Systemically administered dopamine cannot penetrate the 'blood–brain barrier' and is therefore of no benefit   **18.19**

(c) **F** Levodopa produces postural hypotension in about 20% of patients, presumably as a result of interference with central mechanisms controlling blood pressure   **18.21**

(d) **T** In high doses (as an antihypertensive) α-methyldopa may produce Parkinsonism in normal subjects, but in some patients with the disease it may produce beneficial effects   **18.24**

(e) **T** Hypokinesia and rigidity are usually more affected than tremor; amantidine inhibits the uptake of dopamine by dopaminergic neurones and in large doses causes its release — these effects may contribute to its action in Parkinsonism   **18.22**

A287 (a) **F** Since the phenothiazines block dopamine receptors, L-dopa is relatively ineffective; under these conditions the atropine-like drugs are most effective   **18.24**

(b) **T** With reduced dopamine activity there is concurrent excessive cholinergic activity in the corpus striatum which gives rise to abnormal muscle control — thus atropine-like drugs are of benefit   **18.18**

(c) **F** This is a dangerous combination because the cardiac effects of the amphetamine (sympathomimetic) will occur in the presence of vagal cardiac block   **18.23**

(d) **T** The mechanism behind the vasodilator action of dopamine is unclear. However, for whatever reason, postural hypotension occurs in about 20% of patients taking L-dopa   **18.21, 11.27**

(e) **T** When given in combination, the dose of each required is less than when given singly and hence the side-effects are less   **18.21**

Q288 Topical application to the conjunctival surface:

(a) of a substance in a hypertonic solution leads to more ready absorption than from an isotonic solution

(b) of a drug in the ionized form produces rapid absorption

(c) of lignocaine may be used to produce corneal anaesthesia

(d) of idoxuridine may be used to treat viral infections of the cornea

(e) of chloramphenicol may be used to treat bacterial infections of the cornea

Q289 In the eye of normal man:

(a) stimulation of α-adrenoceptors causes pupilloconstriction

(b) stimulation of muscarinic receptors causes pupilloconstriction

(c) stimulation of muscarinic receptors causes a reduction in the near point

(d) there would be dilatation of the pupils in response to a systemic overdose of morphine

(e) the pupil constricts when the gaze moves from far to near objects

Q290 In the eye of normal man:

(a) the protein concentration in the aqueous humour is about the same as in plasma

(b) aqueous humour is formed at a rate of about 3 ml/day

(c) the intraocular pressure is about 50 mmHg

(d) the rate of formation of aqueous humour is directly related to intraocular pressure

(e) intraocular pressure would fall if blood flow to the eye was reduced

A288 (a) F   Drug absorption from hypertonic solution is impaired   **29.4**
due to the osmotic flux of water from the surface of the
eye into the solution

(b) F   The corneal epithelium is most readily penetrated by   **29.4**
non-polar drugs and by non-ionized drug molecules,
since the presence of charge retards movement

(c) T   Lignocaine (lidocaine) in a strength of 4% produces   **20.4**
anaesthesia lasting more than 4 h

(d) T   It is effective against herpes simplex infection of the   **29.4**
cornea because it interferes with viral replication
(blocking incorporation of uridine into DNA)

(e) T   This drug penetrates well into the conjunctival and   **29.6**
corneal epithelium; used topically it does not produce
aplastic anaemia, seen with systemic use

A289 (a) F α-adrenoceptor activation causes contraction of the   **29.8**
dilator pupillae (radial smooth muscle) and hence
mydriasis (i.e. pupil dilatation)

(b) T   Muscarinic activation causes contraction of the   **29.8**
sphincter pupillae (concentric smooth muscle) and hence
miosis

(c) T   Muscarinic activation causes ciliary muscle contrac-   **29.9**
tion, taking the tension off the suspensory ligaments; the
lens grows fatter and its focal length decreases

(d) F   The miotic effect of systemic morphine is partly due to   **29.8**
enhancement of the pupillary light reflex but also to
stimulation of parasympathetic preganglionic cell
bodies in the Edinger-Westphal nucleus

(e) T   This convergence reflex diminishes the spherical and   **29.8**
chromatic aberration of the lens, and increases depth of
focus

A290 (a) F   Aqueous humour is largely formed by ultra-filtration of   **29.9**
plasma, thus its protein concentration is about 5% that
of plasma

(b) T   Equivalent to 2 μl/min which corresponds to a turnover   **29.9**
rate of about 0.6% of the total vol/min

(c) F   The mean pressure is about 15.5 mmHg (range 10–21   **29.10**
mmHg) and is determined principally by the rates of formation and resorption of aqueous humour

(d) F   The filtration from plasma into the anterior chamber is   **29.9**
opposed by the positive intraocular pressure

(e) T   A reduction in blood flow would reduce the rate of   **29.10**
formation of aqueous humour and the intraocular
pressure would fall to a level determined by venous (i.e.
outflow) pressure

Q291 Elevated intraocular pressure:

(a) may result from topical application of glucocorticoids to the conjunctiva

(b) may result from topical application of parasympathomimetics to the conjunctiva

(c) may be reduced by intravenous administration of mannitol

(d) may result from systemic treatment with carbonic anhydrase inhibitors

(e) may be reduced by sympathomimetic amines which penetrate the cornea

Q292 In the retina of normal man:

(a) the photoreceptors called cones are responsible for the detection of colour

(b) the photoreceptors called rods are most densely packed in the region of the fovea centralis

(c) bipolar cells synapse with photoreceptors and ganglion cells

(d) rods contain high levels of rhodopsin in the light-adapted eye

(e) incident photons cause hyperpolarization of rods

A291 (a) **T** Glucocorticoids in 'responders' apparently change the   29.10
glycoprotein of the trabecular tissue in the filtration
angle and reduce the diffusion of aqueous humour

     (b) **F** Pupilloconstriction in response to parasympathomime-   29.12
tics widens the filtration angle and increases the resorption of aqueous humour, hence reducing intraocular
pressure

     (c) **T** Mannitol increases plasma osmotic pressure relative to   29.11
the aqueous humour and hence reduces its formation

     (d) **F** Carbonic anhydrase inhibitors reduce the formation of   29.11
aqueous humour (and hence intraocular pressure) by
impairing active secretion

     (e) **T** Within the eyeball such drugs cause pupilloconstric-   29.14
tion, facilitating resorption of aqueous humour, and
also vasoconstriction, reducing formation of aqueous
humour

A292 (a) **T** In bright light the detection of colour is attributable to   29.23
activation of red/blue/green cones that are sensitive to
the corresponding wavelengths of incident light

     (b) **F** Rods (responsible for vision in dim illumination and   29.23
insensitive to differences in wavelength) do not occur in
the fovea

     (c) **T** The bipolar cells transmit information from rods or   29.23
cones to ganglion cells; they usually have an excitatory
effect on the latter

     (d) **F** On exposure to light the rhodopsin is decomposed;   29.24
pigment cells contain high levels of retinol (vitamin A_1)
and there are minimal amounts of rhodopsin in the rods

     (e) **T** In the dark, the outer segment is permeable to Na^+ 29.25
which is pumped out of the inner segment; on stimulation
Na^+ permeability of the outer segment falls and the cell
hyperpolarizes as Na^+ is pumped out

Metabolism and Nutrition

Q293 In the human subject:

    (a)   resting metabolic rate (per unit body size) is highest at birth

    (b)   thyroxine increases metabolic rate

    (c)   metabolic rate is increased more by intake of protein than by fat

    (d)   metabolic rate is increased by a rise in body temperature

    (e)   shivering is less efficient than co-ordinated muscular activity as a means of maintaining body temperature in the cold

Q294 In Western man, factors influencing heat balance include:

    (a)   radiation, which accounts for about 80% of heat loss

    (b)   the rate of blood flow through cutaneous arterio-venous (a-v) anastomoses

    (c)   loss of heat by evaporation of body water during breathing

    (d)   the thermal conductivity and specific heat of the surrounding medium

    (e)   the rate of evaporation of sweat

A293 (a) **F** The neonate has a metabolic rate of about 16 kJ/h. By 14   **31.3**
days after birth this figure doubles and thereafter
gradually increases over the next few months; subsequently it falls progressively with age

    (b) **T** The effect takes about 2 days to develop and is asso-   **31.3**
ciated with an increase in size and number of mito-
chondria (especially in heart and liver cells) and a dis-
proportionate increase in some enzymes

    (c) **T** Following ingestion of carbohydrate or fat, 5–10% of the   **31.3**
energy content is released as heat; with protein as much
as 40% of its calorific value appears as heat. It has been
suggested that this is a means of regulating body weight,
i.e. 'burning off' calories that are surplus

    (d) **T** For every 1 °C change in body temperature, the meta-   **31.3**
bolic rate changes by about 20%

    (e) **F** Shivering is not accompanied by cutaneous vasodilata-   **31.4**
tion or sweating, but is associated with increased muscle
blood flow. Thus the heat generated acts more effectively to maintain body temperature

A294 (a) **F** Radiation accounts for about 50% of the heat loss (in a   **31.4**
thermoneutral environment) from a naked subject who is
neither sweating nor shivering and when there are no
draughts. The proportion is much less under other conditions

    (b) **T** Rapid blood flow through cutaneous a-v anastomoses   **31.5**
causes less heat to be lost (or gained) by conduction and
convection. Constriction of anastomoses increases
capillary flow, and hence heat exchange

    (c) **T** The amount of heat lost by this route depends on the tem-   **31.5**
perature of the inspired air; it averages about 850 kJ/day
in man. Dogs use this mechanism of thermoregulation (by
panting) so it is of greater importance to them

    (d) **T** Heat loss (or gain) is much more rapid in water than in   **31.5**
air because the thermal conductivity and specific heat of
water is much greater

    (e) **T** It is only when the fluid evaporates that the process of   **31.5**
sweating causes heat loss. Thus sweat not evaporated
(due to high ambient humidity or high sweat rates) does
not contribute to body cooling

Q295 Eccrine sweat gland activity in man:

(a) is inhibited by muscarinic agonists
(b) gives rise to the loss of a hypertonic fluid
(c) can cause marked depletion of total body potassium
(d) can cause serious calcium depletion
(e) is inhibited by atropine-like drugs

Q296 Thermoregulation in man:

(a) is entirely dependent on afferent input from skin hot and cold thermoreceptors
(b) in a cold environment may involve increased lipolysis and glycogenolysis
(c) under normal conditions is impaired by antipyretic drugs
(d) may involve increased circulating levels of corticosteroids
(e) in a hot environment may lead, chronically, to an increased circulating blood volume

A295 (a) **F** In man, eccrine sweat glands have a sympathetic cholinergic excitatory innervation; muscarinic agonists such as pilocarpine cause sweating   **31.5**

(b) **F** Sweat is hypotonic, the main constituent being sodium chloride; the amount of the latter present depends on circulating aldosterone levels   **31.6**

(c) **F** The loss of K^+ (about 9 mmol/l) in sweat does not constitute a serious threat to K^+ balance.   **31.6**

(d) **T** With marked and prolonged sweating, calcium concentration in sweat may rise to 5 mmol/l; with sweat rates of 1.5–4 l/h this can cause hypocalcaemia, with its consequent disturbance of neuromuscular function   **31.6**

(e) **T** Experimentally, and in the treatment of hyperhidrosis (excessive sweating), muscarinic antagonists are effective in inhibiting sweating   **31.6**

A296 (a) **F** Although skin hot and cold thermoreceptors provide important information, this is integrated with the activity of the hypothalamic thermoreceptors   **31.7**

(b) **T** In the short-term these metabolic effects are mediated via circulating adrenaline from the adrenal medulla; both fatty acids and glucose generate increased amounts of metabolic heat and also provide substrate for shivering muscles   **31.8**

(c) **F** Antipyretics only influence thermoregulatory mechanisms in the presence of fever. It is thought that pyrogens enhance the synthesis and release of prostaglandins in the hypothalamus and that antipyretics act by inhibiting prostaglandin synthetase   **31.10**

(d) **T** In the long-term adaptation to cold, the hypothalamic thermostat triggers release of corticotrophin-releasing factor. The resulting elevated steroids in plasma contribute to the drive to increased metabolism in liver and other tissues   **31.14**

(e) **T** Initially blood volume may contract due to excessive sweating, and the filling of the vascular compartment is also compromised by cutaneous vasodilatation. Chronically the volume 'control' mechanisms expand extracellular fluid volume to adapt to this situation   **31.15**

Q297 In a normal adult European male:

(a) the daily energy requirement for average activity is about 12.6 MJ (3000 kcal)

(b) the daily protein intake should be 2 g/kg body weight

(c) the daily intake of essential amino acids is largely derived from vegetables

(d) a carbohydrate-free diet impairs fat metabolism

(e) dietary fat is essential for normal vitamin balance

Q298 In man, vitamin(s):

(a) A deficiency may give rise to corneal abnormalities

(b) D is only obtained from dairy produce

(c) E may be obtained from dairy produce

(d) of the B complex may be obtained from dairy produce

(e) C is synthesized from glucose

A297 (a) **T** Children and the elderly require less; women require slightly less even when doing similar work. The total requirement might typically be met by 70 g protein (1.2 MJ), 100 g fat (3.7 MJ) and 480 g carbohydrate (7.7 MJ)   **43.2**

(b) **F** The recommended daily intake in the UK is 1 g/kg body weight, but it is generally agreed that the minimum requirement for good quality protein is probably less than 0.5 g/kg body weight daily   **43.3**

(c) **F** Most vegetables are low in essential amino acids; these compounds are usually obtained from meat, fish, eggs or milk   **43.3**

(d) **T** Although adaptation to diets very low in carbohydrates is possible, some carbohydrate is essential in order to supply sufficient glycerophosphate to permit fat metabolism to proceed normally, and to avoid ketosis   **43.4, 23.6**

(e) **T** Although calories may be obtained adequately from protein and carbohydrate, some fat in the diet is indispensable since it is the carrier of the fat-soluble vitamins A, D, E and K. Furthermore, linoleic and arachidonic acids can be considered essential polyunsaturated fatty acids (vitaminoids). They are concerned in the formation of cell membranes, membrane transport of fatty acids, mitochondrial metabolism and prostaglandin synthesis   **43.4**

A298 (a) **T** Although the earliest sign of deficiency is impaired dark adaptation (due to reduced amounts of visual pigment in rods), subsequent epithelial dysfunction may cause the cornea to become opaque and soft (keratomalacia), leading to blindness   **43.7**

(b) **F** D vitamins are formed in the skin by ultraviolet (UV) irradiation of steroid precursors (provitamins). Calciferol arises from ergosterol, cholecalciferol from 7-dehydroergosterol and vitamin D_4 from 22, 23-dihydroergosterol. D vitamins formed in the skin are rapidly absorbed into the blood and transported to other sites   **43.8**

(c) **T** E vitamins (tocopherols) occur in the oils from soya bean, wheat germ, rice germ, cotton seed, nuts, maize, butter, eggs, liver and in green leaves   **43.9**

(d) **F** Vitamins of the B complex occur in meats, wholemeal flour, peas, beans and, particularly, yeast   **43.10**

(e) **F** Man, other primates and guinea pigs lack one of the enzymes (L-gulonolactone oxidase) involved in the synthesis of ascorbic acid from glucose. Both L-ascorbic and L-dehydroascorbic acid are present in green plants, tomatoes, citrous fruits, potatoes and in smaller amounts in animal products   **43.15**

Q299 In man, vitamin:

(a) A is obtained entirely from dietary sources

(b) D absorption requires the presence of bile acids

(c) D decreases the absorption of dietary calcium

(d) D has an action of rapid onset

(e) K deficiency may lead to increased coagulability of the blood

Q300 In man, vitamin:

(a) B_1 (thiamine) is most readily obtained from dairy produce

(b) B_1 (thiamine) deficiency is associated with skeletal bone disorders

(c) B_1 (thiamine) is converted into a coenzyme that is involved in carbohydrate metabolism

(d) B_6 deficiency occurs commonly in Third World countries

(e) B_{12} (cyanocobalamin) deficiency may occur after gastrectomy

A299 (a) **T**   Although retinol (vitamin A_1) can be formed in the body,   **43.6**
it is so from carotene precursors (especially β-carotene)
which are pigments present in many fruits and vegetables — particularly carrots and tomatoes. In Britain
about half the dietary vitamin A is derived from precursors in fruit and vegetables

     (b) **T**   Vitamins of the D complex are fat soluble and are   **43.7**
absorbed in the upper part of the small intestine in the
presence of bile acids. Partial esterification occurs
during absorption and the product is transported with
chylomicrons into the lymphatics. In the blood the
vitamin is bound to α_2 globulins and albumin

     (c) **F**   Vitamin D increases the absorption of dietary calcium   **43.8**
(and probably magnesium) and increases the release of
calcium from bone. These effects act to raise plasma calcium levels

     (d) **F**   Vitamin D has an action of slow onset (with a latency of   **43.8**
12–24 h after administration). The delay is partly due to
metabolism of the compound into more active derivatives
and partly to protein synthesis necessary to produce the
effects

     (e) **F**   Vitamin K deficiency leads to hypoprothrombinaemia   **21.8**
(due to decreased synthesis; levels of factors VII, IX and
X are also low), a prolonged one-stage prothrombin time,
and an increased tendency to bleed

A300 (a) **F**   Thiamine is water soluble rather than fat soluble, and is   **43.11**
thus absent from dairy produce. Good sources include
pork, liver, kidneys, whole cereal grains, peas, beans
and yeast

     (b) **F**   Thiamine deficiency gives rise to cardiac failure and   **43.11**
oedema; thiamine deficiency associated with lack of
additional B vitamins gives rise to peripheral neuritis,
wasting and partial paralysis

     (c) **T**   Thiamine is converted into thiamine pyrophosphate in   **43.11**
the intestinal mucosa; this acts as a coenzyme in the
oxidative decarboxylation of pyruvate and α-oxoglu-
tarate in the Krebs' cycle, and in many other reactions

     (d) **F**   Most diets contain adequate amounts and some is   **43.12**
synthesized by intestinal flora. Pyridoxine is plentiful in
vegetables and pyridoxamine and pyridoxal in animal
matter; the three forms are interconvertible in the body

     (e) **T**   Absorption of dietary vitamin B_{12} depends on the forma-   **21.37**
tion of a complex with a glycoprotein (intrinsic factor)
secreted by the parietal cells of the gastric mucosa

Endocrines

Q301 In the pituitary gland:

(a) the anterior and posterior lobes are derived from a single embryological origin
(b) the posterior lobe contains large amounts of neural tissue
(c) the posterior lobe controls the output of several other endocrine glands
(d) the anterior lobe is highly vascular
(e) the anterior lobe is sparsely innervated

Q302 In the anterior lobe of the pituitary:

(a) the cells are differentiated into two main types
(b) chromophobes contain large dense granules
(c) 50% of the cells are chromophils in normal man
(d) the basophils secrete growth hormone and prolactin
(e) corticotrophin is secreted by chromophobes

Q303 Hypophysiotrophic hormones:

(a) are secreted by neurones in the median eminence of the hypothalamus
(b) are transported through the hypophyseal portal system to the posterior pituitary
(c) act on target cells to stimulate the release of hormones
(d) may act by stimulating adenylate cyclase
(e) are under the control of monoamine neurotransmitters in the hypothalamus

A301   (a)   **F**   The posterior lobe is derived from a downward projection of the floor of the third ventricle; the anterior lobe is derived from the ectodermal layer of the dorsal pharynx (Rathke's pouch)   **19.2**

       (b)   **T**   The posterior lobe contains nerve endings and neuroglial cells   **19.2**

       (c)   **F**   Trophic hormones from the *anterior* lobe control the output from the thyroid, adrenal, ovary and testis   **19.1**

       (d)   **T**   The cords of cells which form the anterior lobe have numerous vascular sinusoids between them   **19.3**

       (e)   **T**   The only innervation in the anterior lobe is a sympathetic supply to the larger blood vessels   **19.3**

A302   (a)   **T**   This distinction (chromophils and chromophobes) is made on the basis of their appearance after different histological staining procedures   **19.3**

       (b)   **F**   Chromophobes are agranular and are probably precursors of chromophils; chromophils are granular   **19.3**

       (c)   **T**   Of the chromophils, about 35% are acidophils and 15% are basophils   **19.3**

       (d)   **F**   Acidophils secrete growth hormone (500 μg/day) and prolactin; basophils secrete follicle-stimulating hormone, luteinizing hormone, thyrotrophin and melanocyte-stimulating hormone   **19.3**

       (e)   **T**   Corticotrophin (ACTH) appears to be the only hormone secreted by this cell type; secretion rate is normally about 10 μg/day   **19.3**

A303   (a)   **T**   Neurones called neuroendocrine transducers in the arcuate and other nuclei secrete these hormones   **19.5**

       (b)   **F**   The portal system begins as a network of capillaries in the ventral hypothalamus and ends in capillaries associated with the *anterior* lobe of the pituitary   **19.5**

       (c)   **F**   Of the 9 hypophysiotrophic hormones so far identified in man, 6 stimulate release whilst 3 inhibit release of anterior pituitary hormones   **19.5**

       (d)   **T**   Stimulation of adenylate cyclase and production of cyclic AMP mediates the action of at least some hypophysiotrophic hormones   **19.5**

       (e)   **T**   Dopamine, noradrenaline and serotonin-containing neurones impinge on the neuroendocrine transducer cells and influence hormone release   **19.5, 19.6**

Q304 Human growth hormone:

    (a)   is under the control of hypothalamic stimulatory and inhibitory factors

    (b)   reduces hepatic glucose release

    (c)   antagonizes the action of insulin on glucose uptake

    (d)   promotes the secretion of somatomedins from the liver and kidney

    (e)   is secreted in response to insulin-induced hypoglycaemia

Q305 In man, growth hormone:

    (a)   elevates blood glucose

    (b)   has a direct stimulant effect on the sulphation of cartilage

    (c)   release during exercise is inhibited by propranolol

    (d)   production is normal in most types of dwarfism

    (e)   release is reduced in hypothyroidism

A304 (a) **T** Growth-hormone-releasing hormone and growth-hormone-release-inhibiting hormone (somatostatin) control secretion   **19.5, 19.8**

(b) **F** Growth hormone increases release of glucose from the liver and reduces glucose uptake by some tissues   **19.7**

(c) **T** This effect of growth hormone together with the influence on hepatic glucose release can produce diabetes mellitus in cases of oversecretion   **19.7**

(d) **T** Somatomedins A and B (growth-hormone-dependent factors) stimulate DNA synthesis in several tissues and thus promote cell division   **19.8**

(e) **T** The release of growth hormone in response to a fall in blood glucose (below 2.2 mmol/l) is sometimes used as a diagnostic test of pituitary function   **19.8**

A305 (a) **T** Growth hormone decreases the uptake of glucose by some tissues and increases hepatic glucose release. The elevation of blood glucose promotes insulin release, but growth hormone inhibits the action of insulin on skeletal muscle. Somatomedins released from the liver in response to growth hormone have an insulin-like effect. So the elevation in blood glucose is an outcome of the interaction between all these factors   **19.7**

(b) **F** Although growth hormone causes proliferation of cartilage (as reflected by increased hydroxyproline turnover) associated with an increase in the length of long bones, this effect is indirect   **19.7**

(c) **F** Growth hormone is released in response to exercise and hypoglycaemia; in both situations propranolol (a non-selective β-adrenoceptor antagonist) enhances release. It is possible that this effect is due to inhibition of somatostatin release   **19.8**

(d) **T** Failure to grow in the presence of normal plasma levels of growth hormone may be due to end-organ resistance, the production of a biologically (but not immunologically) inactive form of the hormone, or the failure to elaborate somatomedins in response to growth hormone   **19.9**

(e) **T** There is a decrease in synthesis, storage and release of growth hormone in hypothyroidism, as well as a reduction in the direct, growth-promoting effects of thyroid hormones   **19.8**

Q306 Prolactin secretion:

(a) increases during the first trimester of pregnancy
(b) increases in response to suckling of the lactating breast
(c) would fall following destruction of the hypothalamus
(d) falls in response to an elevation in hypothalamic dopamine
(e) in the non-pregnant adult shows a circadian rhythm with peak values in the early morning

Q307 In human subjects:

(a) prolactin has important direct effects on renal function
(b) chlorpromazine causes an increase in plasma prolactin levels
(c) bromocriptine may be used in treating hypoprolactinaemia
(d) chronic corticosteroid therapy increases skin pigmentation
(e) melatonin has no effect on skin pigmentation

Q308 In the posterior lobe of the pituitary:

(a) there are nerve terminals which have cell bodies in the hypothalamus
(b) the hormones oxytocin and vasopressin are stored in nerve endings
(c) stored hormones are bound to a single protein known as neurophysin
(d) hormone release is stimulated by magnesium
(e) hormones are released directly into capillaries

A306 (a) **F** Prolactin secretion rises only during the last month of pregnancy — 19.9

(b) **T** The episodic reflex stimulation of the breast by suckling releases prolactin which maintains the gland in an actively lactating state — 19.10

(c) **F** Prolactin release is under the influence of an inhibitory hormone from the hypothalamus; removal of this influence promotes release — 19.10

(d) **T** The hypothalamic prolactin-release-inhibiting hormone is probably dopamine — 19.10

(e) **T** The circadian rhythm is seen in both sexes, but disappears in pregnancy — 19.9

A307 (a) **F** Although there is some evidence that prolactin has anti-natriuretic and anti-diuretic effects, these are probably secondary to changes in plasma aldosterone and ADH levels — 19.10

(b) **T** Prolactin release is under the influence of a release-inhibiting hormone which itself is controlled by hypothalamic dopamine. Drugs which antagonize dopamine receptors (such as chlorpromazine [**15.5**]) thus reduce the inhibitory influence, and prolactin release is increased — 19.10

(c) **F** Bromocriptine (an ergot-alkaloid derivative) stimulates central dopamine receptors and hence suppresses prolactin secretion; it is thus used to treat hyperprolactinaemia (in women the latter causes galactorrhoea, in men gynaecomastia and impotence) — 19.10

(d) **F** Exogenous steroids suppress release of adrenocorticotrophic hormone and melanocyte-stimulating hormone, thus skin pigmentation is reduced — 32.13

(e) **T** In animals with melanophores, melatonin inhibits the action of melanocyte-stimulating hormone, and thus causes lightening of the skin. In man, melatonin may play an inhibitory role on sexual development during puberty — 19.11, 32.12

A308 (a) **T** The cell bodies are in the paraventricular and supra-optic nuclei of the anterior hypothalamus — 19.12

(b) **T** Secretory granules composed of hormone plus neurophysin are transported from the hypothalamus and stored in the posterior pituitary — 19.13

(c) **F** There are two neurophysins; in the hypothalamus oxytocin is always combined with neurophysin I and vasopressin with neurophysin II — 19.13

(d) **F** Ionized calcium is necessary for release and magnesium antagonizes the action of calcium — 19.13

(e) **T** In this way the process differs from transmitter release from neurones generally, where the substance is released into a junctional cleft — 19.13

Q309 Vasopressin (antidiuretic hormone):

(a) release is stimulated by a reduction in plasma osmolality

(b) release is stimulated by a reduction in circulating blood volume

(c) acts in the kidney to reduce water reabsorption

(d) is a powerful vasoconstrictor

(e) deficiency is characterized by polydipsia and polyuria

Q310 In man, polyuria:

(a) may be due to a lack of antidiuretic hormone (primary idiopathic diabetes insipidus)

(b) may occur when plasma antidiuretic hormone levels are high

(c) may be due to high circulating ethanol levels

(d) due to nephrogenic diabetes insipidus may be treated with thiazide diuretics

(e) due to nephrogenic diabetes insipidus may be treated with chlorpropamide

A309 (a) **F** An *increase* in plasma osmolality is sensed by osmo- 19.13
receptors in or near the supraoptic and paraventricular
nuclei and stimulates vasopressin release

(b) **T** Volume depletion such as haemorrhage is a potent 19.14
stimulus for vasopressin release (this effect is mediated
through cardiopulmonary and arterial baroreceptors)

(c) **F** Vasopressin acts on the collecting duct to increase water 19.13
reabsorption by enhancing the permeability of the duct
to water

(d) **T** Although the concentration of vasopressin required to 19.14
produce an increase in blood pressure is far greater
than that required to produce maximal antidiuresis, it
does have marked vasoconstrictor effects in certain vascular beds

(e) **T** This condition is known as diabetes insipidus; the 19.15
inability to reabsorb water results in large quantities of
hypotonic urine being produced. Increased plasma
osmolality and reduced plasma volume stimulate thirst

A310 (a) **T** This rare disorder gives rise to polydipsia and polyuria 19.14
(usually 5–10 l/day), and is attributable to failure to
elaborate antidiuretic hormone

(b) **T** In nephrogenic diabetes insipidus renal tubular cells 19.14,
become unresponsive to antidiuretic hormone. This can 19.35
happen in chronic hypokalaemia and following lithium
therapy

(c) **T** Ethanol has a marked inhibitory effect on antidiuretic 19.15
hormone release. Thus the diuresis is not simply due to a
large volume intake (e.g. if beer is being drunk) and can
result in marked dehydration

(d) **T** Thiazides appear to cause redistribution of body sodium 19.14
and reduction of ECF volume. This activates sodium-
retaining (proximal tubular) forces and hence increases
water reabsorption

(e) **F** Chlorpropamide is only beneficial in primary idiopathic 19.15
(neurogenic) diabetes insipidus. The mechanism of this
action is unclear. One possibility is that chlorpropamide
potentiates the antidiuretic effect of small circulating
amounts of vasopressin

Q311 Oxytocin:

(a) release is stimulated by stretch receptors in the vagina

(b) produces more powerful uterine contractions in the presence of high circulating progesterone levels

(c) secretion rate increases during late pregnancy

(d) promotes milk ejection

(e) is synthesized mainly in cell bodies of the paraventricular nucleus

Q312 In man the thyroid gland:

(a) produces only two hormones, thyroxine and tri-iodothyronine

(b) is unique among endocrine glands in that the thyroid hormones are stored extracellularly

(c) contains numerous follicles (acini) which are swollen with colloid when active

(d) contains cells known as parafollicular cells

(e) develops as an outgrowth of endodermal tissue from the floor of the pharynx

A311 (a) **T** At birth, the descent of the fetus stimulates stretch receptors in the uterus and vagina and thus initiates oxytocin release   **19.14**

(b) **F** The action of oxytocin is intensified by oestrogens and weakened by progesterone   **20.54**

(c) **F** Oxytocin secretion increases during the early stages of pregnancy after which it remains at a constant elevated level   **20.54**

(d) **T** By causing contraction of the myoepithelial cells of the alveolar ducts oxytocin causes and maintains milk release   **19.12, 20.16**

(e) **F** Oxytocin is largely manufactured in the cell bodies of the supraoptic nucleus. The paraventricular nucleus synthesizes vasopressin predominantly   **19.13**

A312 (a) **F** The thyroid gland also produces calcitonin — a polypeptide hormone involved in the regulation of plasma calcium concentration   **19.16**

(b) **T** This is in the form of colloid in the acinar lumen   **19.16**

(c) **F** When the follicles are actively synthesizing and secreting hormones the colloid is broken down by proteases   **19.17**

(d) **T** These cells (also known as C cells) produce calcitonin. In lower vertebrates they form a discrete structure called the ultimobranchial body   **19.16**

(e) **T** This occurs in association with the formation of the parathyroid glands which develop from the third and fourth pharyngeal pouches   **19.16**

Q313 In the human thyroid gland:

    (a)   iodide ions from plasma enter the follicle cells by passive diffusion

    (b)   sequestration of iodide takes place by a process unique to this tissue

    (c)   thyroxine, once synthesized, is then coupled to thyroglobulin until released

    (d)   a greater proportion of tri-iodothyronine is formed when iodine is deficient

    (e)   which is actively secreting, the acini contain large amounts of colloid

Q314 Thyroxine:

    (a)   production involves uptake of iodide from the plasma by diffusion

    (b)   in plasma is largely protein bound

    (c)   is metabolized by the liver

    (d)   production involves iodination of tyramine

    (e)   has more potent hormonal effects than tri-iodothyronine

A313 (a) **F**   Treatment with drugs that block the incorporation of   **19.17**
iodine into protein, but do not interfere with the uptake
of iodide by the follicular cells, reveals that the follicular
cells can accumulate iodide against a concentration
gradient of 250:1 (plasma levels are about 3 μg/l)

    (b)   **F**   The existence of active mechanisms for iodide uptake   **19.17**
(similar to that of the follicular cells) has been demon-
strated in salivary and mammary glands and gastric
mucosa. However, TSH has no effect on these processes

    (c)   **F**   Tyrosine (an amino acid) is iodinated when it is linked by   **19.17**
peptide bonds to thyroglobulin (a glycoprotein) contain-
ing about 100 tyrosine residues per molecule

    (d)   **T**   When iodine is scarce, fewer di-iodotyrosyl residues are   **19.19**
formed and the coupling between them (to form
thyroxine) is less likely than coupling between di-iodo-
and mono-iodotyrosyl residues. Since tri-iodothyronine
is more active than thyroxine this maximizes the effect of
the available iodine

    (e)   **F**   In the inactive gland, large amounts of colloid are stored,   **19.17**
and the follicular cells are narrow. In the actively
secreting gland, the follicular cells are columnar, the
acini small and only trace amounts of colloid are found in
them

A314 (a) **F**   Hormone production does involve iodide uptake but this   **19.16**
occurs by an active process against chemical and elec-
trical gradients

    (b)   **T**   Only about 0.05% of the total plasma thyroxine and   **19.19**
0.5–0.75% of the tri-iodothyronine is not protein bound

    (c)   **T**   Deiodination, oxidative deamination and conjugation   **19.19**
with glucuronic and sulphuric acids are the principle
metabolic processes

    (d)   **F**   *Tyrosine* residues attached to thyroglobulin are   **19.17**
iodinated in the process of thyroid hormone production

    (e)   **F**   The hormonal effects of tri-iodothyronine are more   **19.19**
marked and rapid in onset than those of thyroxine.
Furthermore, tri-iodothyronine is less tightly bound to
plasma proteins, so the plasma levels of the free
hormones are similar (even though the absolute amount
of tri-iodothyronine is much less)

Q315 In the human, the thyroid hormone thyroxine:

    (a)   has a half-life of about 2 days

    (b)   undergoes enterohepatic recirculation

    (c)   increases the oxygen consumption of brain tissue

    (d)   increases glucose absorption from the gastrointestinal tract

    (e)   in excess, causes suppression of the sympathoadrenal system

Q316 In normal man:

    (a)   thyroxine causes an immediate increase in oxygen consumption and metabolic rate

    (b)   thyroxine lowers plasma cholesterol concentration

    (c)   heart rate and systolic blood pressure increase in response to thyroxine administered intravenously

    (d)   thyroid hormones act on the hypothalamus to inhibit the synthesis of thyrotrophin-releasing hormone (TRH)

    (e)   thyroid hormones act on the pituitary to inhibit the secretion of thyrotrophin

A315 (a) **F** Thyroxine is extensively protein bound (about 0.05% is free in plasma) to specific proteins (thyroxine-binding globulin or thyroxine-binding pre-albumin) or to plasma albumin. This leads to a slow turnover, with a half-life of 6–7 days; triiodothyronine which is much less tightly bound has a half-life of about 2 days **19.19**

(b) **T** The metabolism of thyroxine occurs mainly in the liver (although some is converted to tri-iodothyronine by other tissues) by deiodination, oxidative deamination, glucuronidation and sulphation. Some conjugated thyroxine is excreted in the bile, where it is hydrolysed and then reabsorbed **19.19**

(c) **F** Thyroxine (over a period of about 2 days) increases oxygen consumption of heart, gastric mucosa, liver, kidney, smooth and skeletal muscle, but not brain, gonads or reticuloendothelial tissue. The stimulant effect is probably due to increased numbers and size of mitochondria and elevated enzyme activities **19.20**

(d) **T** This effect is probably due to increased mucosal activity subsequent to mitochondrial changes. However, the stimulation of catabolism leads to reduction in hepatic glycogen levels and loss of fat and protein depots **19.20**

(e) **F** Hyperthyroidism is associated with tachycardia, elevated cardiac output, increased oxygen consumption, restlessness and tremor — all features of sympatho-adrenal hyperactivity **19.20**

A316 (a) **F** The calorigenic effect of thyroxine takes about 2 days to reach its maximum **19.20**

(b) **T** This occurs due to increased elimination of cholesterol despite an increased cholesterol synthesis by the liver **19.20, 19.29**

(c) **T** There is some evidence that this may be due to an interaction with the sympathetic nervous system **19.20**

(d) **F** There is a positive feedback input at the hypothalamic level and a negative feedback on to the pituitary **19.21**

(e) **T** The level of TRH secretion is thought to determine the sensitivity of the anterior lobe of the pituitary to the inhibitory influence of thyroxine **19.21**

Q317 In the human subject, thyroid function:

(a) is increased by thyrotrophin, through its binding with nuclear receptors

(b) is enhanced at low environmental temperatures

(c) in Graves' disease (primary hyperthyroidism) is abnormal due to increased production of thyrotrophin by the pituitary

(d) in lymphocytic thyroiditis is abnormal, often due to circulating antibodies to thyroglobulin

(e) is always excessive when goitre is present

Q318 In hyperthyroid states:

(a) retraction of the upper eyelids is common

(b) carbimazole may be given as treatment

(c) large quantities (about 6 mg/day) of iodine exacerbate the disturbance

(d) sympathetic blocking drugs reduce thyroid hormone secretion

(e) intravenously administered TRH fails to cause thyrotrophin release

A317 (a) **F** Thyrotrophin does not enter follicular cells; all its effects **19.21**
are a result of its interaction with the follicular cell mem-
brane, possibly by activation of membrane adenylate
cyclase, leading to increased cyclic AMP production

(b) **T** This is due to increased synthesis and release of TRH. **19.22**
The effect is not likely to be due to changes in levels of
circulating thyroid hormones, but is more likely attributable to enhanced activity of the noradrenergic neurones
that synapse with the TRH neurones

(c) **F** In Graves' disease, TRH levels are usually low due to **19.23**
pituitary suppression by the high circulating levels of
thyroid hormone. It is likely that the hyperthyroidism is
due to thyroid-stimulating substances of extra-pituitary
origin

(d) **T** The disorder is frequently associated with the presence **19.25**
of circulating antibodies to thyroglobulin or another
component of the thyroid tissue. The antigen–antibody
reactions lead to inflammation and lymphocytic infiltra-
tion

(e) **F** The depressed thyroid function associated with the use **19.23**
of antithyroid drugs is usually associated with the development of goitre because the reduced levels of thyroid
hormones disinhibit thyrotrophin release and the latter
causes thyroid hyperplasia

A318 (a) **T** This is due to increased tone in the superior palpebral **19.23**
muscle mediated via its noradrenergic innervation (c.f.
also resting tachycardia due to sympathetic hyperactivity)

(b) **T** This drug (a thiocarbamide) interferes with iodide bind- **19.24**
ing by the thyroid glands and hence with thyroid
hormone synthesis

(c) **F** Paradoxically, in large quantities, iodine given to a **19.25**
hyperthyroid person reduces the thyroid gland secre-
tion; the effect is rapid but the mechanism unknown

(d) **F** Sympathetic blocking drugs may be given to offset some **19.25**
of the symptoms (e.g. tachycardia) but they do not reduce
hormone secretion

(e) **T** In the presence of high circulating thyroxine levels, the **19.28**
sensitivity of the anterior pituitary to TRH is reduced

Q319 In hypothyroid states:

(a) the size of the thyroid gland is always subnormal
(b) the uptake of radioactive iodide by the thyroid gland is low
(c) injection of thyroxine distinguishes primary and secondary disturbances
(d) basal metabolic rate is low
(e) plasma lipid levels are elevated

Q320 The production of thyroid hormones:

(a) may be reduced by thiocyanates which inhibit the organic binding of iodine
(b) is usually increased in patients treated with lithium
(c) may be reduced by guanethidine or propranolol
(d) is not stimulated by TRH in hypothyroidism due to hypopituitarism
(e) may be reduced by drugs of the thiocarbamide group, such as carbimazole

A319 (a) **F** If, for instance, the hypothyroidism is due to excessive treatment with antithyroid drugs, the reduced circulating hormone levels facilitate increased thyrotrophin release which results in hyperplasia of the thyroid gland   **19.23**

(b) **T** This is used in the diagnosis of thyroid dysfunction; the uptake of ^{131}I is related to the rate of thyroid hormone secretion   **19.28**

(c) **F** Injection of thyrotrophin distinguishes primary hypothyroidism (insufficient functional thyroid tissue) from secondary hypothyroidism due to a pituitary disturbance   **19.25**

(d) **T** It may be as much as 30 to 40% below normal. Although the reason for this is unclear it is possible that the effect is due to diminished mitochondrial size and permeability   **19.25**

(e) **T** The effect of thyroxine to enhance elimination of cholesterol is greater than its stimulatory effect on hepatic cholesterol synthesis   **19.20**

A320 (a) **F** Perchlorates, fluoroborates, thiocyanates and nitrates inhibit synthesis of thyroid hormones by competing with iodide for uptake by the follicular cells   **19.23**

(b) **F** Although in some patients treated with lithium, goitre has been reported to develop, they remain euthyroid and the condition is reversible. The explanation of the effect is not known   **19.27**

(c) **F** These drugs serve to inhibit the sympathoadrenal hyperactivity (or its effects) seen in thyrotoxicosis. They do not reduce the production of thyroid hormones   **19.25**

(d) **T** In this condition injection of thyrotrophin leads to increased uptake of iodine by the thyroid glands, but TRH fails to have an effect becaue the thyrotrophs of the anterior pituitary are defective   **19.25**

(e) **T** Drugs such as carbimazole probably act by sequestering a reactive intermediary compound (possibly sulphenyl iodide), thereby interfering with the iodination of tyrosine. However, there is some evidence that these drugs may have a selective effect on the coupling reaction   **19.24**

Q321 In the adrenal glands:

(a) there is an inner medulla and outer cortex which differ in their embryological development
(b) both cortex and medulla are richly innervated
(c) the medulla and cortex have separate blood supplies
(d) the hormones produced in the cortex pass directly to the medulla
(e) adrenaline synthesis may be decreased in pituitary deficiency

Q322 In normal man:

(a) the mean plasma concentrations of cortisol and aldosterone are similar
(b) cortisol is the predominant glucocorticoid hormone
(c) cortisol does not significantly contribute to mineralo-corticoid activity
(d) aldosterone contributes to glucocorticoid activity
(e) adrenal steroid hormones have specific effects either on carbohydrate metabolism or on electrolyte and water balance

Q323 The synthesis of adrenal steroids:

(a) begins with a common precursor, cholesterol
(b) is impaired by drugs used clinically to lower plasma cholesterol concentration
(c) involves removal of part of the side-chain of cholesterol to form progesterone
(d) is antagonized by inhibitors of protein synthesis such as cycloheximide
(e) may be impaired by tricyclic antidepressants

A321 (a) **T** The medulla is formed from migratory ectodermal cells   **19.29,**
            from the neural crest. The cortex is of mesodermal   **19.30**
            origin, developing from the coelomic mesothelium

      (b) **F** The medulla is well innervated by preganglionic   **19.29**
            cholinergic fibres but the cortex has a relatively sparse
            innervation, mostly associated with blood vessels

      (c) **F** They have a common blood supply — each gland is sup-   **19.29**
            plied by branches from the phrenic artery, the
            abdominal aorta and the renal artery

      (d) **T** This is achieved by the intra-adrenal portal system. The   **19.29**
            cortical hormones influence the synthesis (and, possibly,
            release) of medullary catecholamines

      (e) **T** Corticotrophin stimulates glucocorticoid secretion; the   **19.36**
            elevated glucocorticoid levels in blood perfusing the
            medulla induces phenylethanolamine-N-methyltrans-
            ferase activity and hence increases adrenaline synthesis
            and vice versa

A322 (a) **F** The mean plasma concentration of cortisol is approxi-   **19.31**
            mately 100 μg/l whereas that of aldosterone is only
            0.1 μg/l

      (b) **T** Cortisol (hydrocortisone) predominates in man (daily   **19.31**
            secretion 15–30 mg) with corticosterone being secreted
            at 2–5 mg per day

      (c) **F** Because of its high concentration and in spite of its weak   **19.31,**
            mineralocorticoid activity, cortisol exerts substantial   **Table**
            mineralocorticoid effects   **19.6**

      (d) **F** Because of its low concentration, despite some weak glu-   **19.31,**
            cocorticoid activity, aldosterone does not exert any   **Table**
            significant glucocorticoid effects   **19.5**

      (e) **F** The glucocorticoids are *relatively* more powerful in   **19.31**
            affecting carbohydrate metabolism; the mineralocorti-
            coids predominantly affect water and electrolyte
            balance

A323 (a) **T** Some of the cholesterol is synthesized and stored within   **19.31**
            the gland, but most is taken up from the plasma

      (b) **F** These drugs produce only a small decrease in the avail-   **19.33**
            ability of cholesterol

      (c) **F** Pregnenolone is formed by removal of part of the side-   **19.31**
            chain from cholesterol

      (d) **T** Drugs which block protein synthesis block steroido-   **19.33,**
            genesis by inhibiting the production of a number of   **19.37**
            enzymes involved in steroid synthesis

      (e) **T** This is an indirect effect due to a reduction in cortico-   **19.33**
            trophin secretion, and is shared with other centrally
            active drugs that may affect hypothalamic neurotrans-
            mitter levels

Q324 In man, a deficiency in 21-β-hydroxylase:

   (a)   causes adrenal hypertrophy
   (b)   reduces the production of hydrocortisone
   (c)   reduces the production of androgens
   (d)   may lead to salt retention
   (e)   increases the formation of deoxycortisol and deoxy-
         corticosterone

Q325 In normal man, glucocorticoids:

   (a)   promote the mobilization of proteins and amino acids
         from skeletal muscle
   (b)   deplete liver glycogen stores
   (c)   stimulate lipolysis directly
   (d)   administered in large doses over a long period of time
         result in hypersensitivity to insulin
   (e)   decrease the number of lymphocytes in the blood

A324 (a) **F** The congenital absence of 21-β-hydroxylase results in adrenal hyperplasia since pituitary corticotrophin release is stimulated   **19.33**

    (b) **T** This deficiency gives rise to reduced synthesis of corticosterone and deoxycortisol, both of which are precursors of hydrocortisone   **19.33**

    (c) **F** There is increased adrenal androgen production since the precursor 17–OH-progesterone is converted into androgens instead of deoxycortisol   **19.33**

    (d) **F** In severe cases there may be salt loss, due to a deficiency in aldosterone production   **19.33**

    (e) **F** These are reduced; it is when 11-β-hydroxylase is deficient that the levels of these substances increase   **19.33**

A325 (a) **T** Proteins and amino acids mobilized from skeletal muscle (and also from bone matrix and skin) then enter the bloodstream and are carried to the liver   **19.34**

    (b) **F** Enzymes involved in glycogenesis are stimulated by glucocorticoids, hence liver glycogen stores increase   **19.34**

    (c) **F** A minimal amount of steroid is necessary before lipolysis can occur in response to hormones such as adrenaline and glucagon, but the steroids themselves have no direct lipolytic activity   **19.34, 19.35**

    (d) **F** The abnormally high blood glucose concentrations which occur cause hyposensitivity to insulin and may produce a diabetic-like state   **19.35**

    (e) **T** Glucocorticoids cause involution of lymphoid tissue and destruction of lymphocytes in the thymus, spleen and lymph nodes; mitosis in the lymphocytes that remain is inhibited   **13.10**

Q326 In normal man:

(a) mineralocorticoids stimulate sodium reabsorption in the distal tubule of the kidney

(b) excess administration of mineralocorticoids over several days causes increasing sodium retention

(c) reduced secretion of aldosterone may cause hyperkalaemia

(d) mineralocorticoids influence the electrolyte composition of saliva

(e) adrenal steroids inhibit adrenaline synthesis

Q327 Corticosteroid binding globulin:

(a) is the only protein fraction involved in the binding of adrenal steroids in plasma

(b) synthesis in the liver is increased by oestrogen

(c) levels in plasma are depressed in nephrosis

(d) excess chronically reduces the concentration of free steroid hormone

(e) has a high affinity and a low total binding capacity

Q328 Corticotrophin (adrenocorticotrophic hormone):

(a) is released from the hypothalamus

(b) activates steroid synthesis via increased production of cyclic AMP

(c) stimulates hydrolysis of cholesterol

(d) stimulates secretion of adrenal steroids

(e) secretion normally shows a diurnal rhythm with lowest levels during sleep

A326	(a)	T	This effect may be due to increased activity of sodium pumps and/or increased numbers of pumps and/or increased membrane permeability to sodium	19.35
	(b)	F	After a few days of mineralocorticoid administration, the sodium retaining effect is lost (possibly due to changes in proximal tubular sodium handling), although the potassium losing effect persists; this phenomenon is known as 'mineralocorticoid escape'	19.35
	(c)	T	The reabsorption of sodium is accompanied by secretion of potassium; reduced aldosterone secretion may thus cause plasma potassium levels to rise	19.35
	(d)	T	Enhanced sodium reabsorption and potassium secretion in response to mineralocorticoids occurs not only in the kidney, but also in salivary glands, sweat glands, the exocrine pancreas and the intestine	19.35
	(e)	F	Adrenal steroids stimulate the synthesis of phenyl-ethanolamine-N-methyltransferase and thereby facilitate the production of adrenaline from noradrenaline	19.36

A327	(a)	F	There are two, the other is plasma albumin	19.36
	(b)	T	This results in elevated concentrations during pregnancy	19.36
	(c)	T	Because of defective filtration in the damaged kidney the binding globulin is lost in the urine	19.36
	(d)	F	A transient reduction in free hormone levels stimulates the release of corticotrophin and a new equilibrium is reached in which the concentration of free hormone remains normal	19.36
	(e)	T	The converse is true for albumin — it has a low affinity but a high binding capacity	19.36

A328	(a)	F	A releasing factor from the hypothalamus controls the release of corticotrophin from the anterior pituitary	19.37, 19.6
	(b)	T	This occurs mostly in the zona fasciculata and zona reticularis of the cortex	19.37
	(c)	T	This is the first step in adrenal steroid synthesis — it results in the formation of pregnenolone	19.37, 19.32
	(d)	T	Since adrenal steroids are not stored to any extent, increased synthesis is accompanied by increased release	19.37
	(e)	F	The peak occurs just before waking and the lowest level is in the late evening	19.38

Q329 Cortisone:

(a) is a naturally occurring steroid secreted by the adrenal glands

(b) is used as a topical corticosteroid in the treatment of dermatitis and eczema

(c) may be given orally or intramuscularly as replacement therapy in Addison's disease

(d) given orally, may reduce the frequency and severity of migraine attacks

(e) may be given orally in the treatment of severe bronchial asthma

Q330 In primary adrenocortical insufficiency:

(a) patients are prone to develop hypoglycaemia

(b) capillary permeability to protein is reduced

(c) the skin may become pigmented

(d) there is a tendency to develop hypokalaemia

(e) patients may become hypotensive

A329 (a) **F**   Cortisone is a metabolite of hydrocortisone — it is not secreted by the adrenals   **19.37**

(b) **T**   The anti-inflammatory and immunosuppressant activity of cortisone depends on its conversion to hydrocortisone   **19.42, 32.21**

(c) **T**   Systemic administration is effective since cortisone is metabolized to hydrocortisone in the liver   **19.42**

(d) **T**   The symptoms of migraine (scalp vasodilatation and oedema, resembling inflammatory responses) may be reduced by repeated administration of cortisone, as may the frequency of attacks   **16.40**

(e) **T**   The mechanism of the beneficial action is poorly understood, but is probably a combination of membrane stabilization, reduced mediator release and enhanced catecholamine action   **19.42, 24.29**

A330 (a) **T**   Glucocorticoids normally promote the synthesis of enzymes involved in gluconeogenesis and glycogenolysis. In insufficiency states, a brief period of starvation rapidly depletes carbohydrate reserves   **19.34, 19.39**

(b) **F**   It is increased, with the result that the distribution of body water and electrolytes is deranged   **19.35**

(c) **T**   This is because the low levels of glucocorticoids disinhibits release of corticotrophin and melanocyte-stimulating hormone   **19.39**

(d) **F**   Due to insufficient potassium secretion, hyperkalaemia develops with consequent abnormalities in the ECG and tissue excitability   **19.35, 19.38**

(e) **T**   This is likely to be due to a combination of an absolute volume depletion (due to renal salt and water loss) and an additional reduction in extracellular fluid volume (due to a shift of fluid into cells)   **19.39, 19.35**

Q331 In adrenocortical hypersecretion:

    (a)   the skin becomes thickened
    (b)   there may be muscle weakness and wasting
    (c)   the bones become hardened
    (d)   metabolic alkalosis may develop
    (e)   polyuria may develop

Q332 The anti-inflammatory action of adrenal steroids:

    (a)   is common to both mineralo- and gluco-corticoids
    (b)   is mediated through suppression of the cellular response to injury only
    (c)   is partly due to their facilitatory action on the effects of circulating catecholamines
    (d)   occurs at normal levels of steroid secretion
    (e)   involves a reduction in histamine release

Q333 In the human pancreas:

    (a)   the cells of the islets of Langerhans derive from the neural crest
    (b)   the blood vessels of the islets drain into the portal vein
    (c)   40% of the islet cells store insulin
    (d)   all the β-cells secrete glucagon
    (e)   the islets are not connected to the pancreatic duct system

A331 (a) **F** The skin is thin and transparent (probably due to reduction of the protein matrix) **19.40**

(b) **T** Excess mineralocorticoids cause muscle weakness (probably due to hypokalaemia); excess glucocorticoids cause muscle wasting (due to protein breakdown) **19.36**

(c) **F** Osteoporosis develops due to **19.40**
    (i)   excess protein catabolism inhibiting new bone formation;
    (ii) glucocorticoids inhibiting the action of vitamin D;
    (iii) glucocorticoids increasing glomerular filtration rate and thus increasing calcium excretion

(d) **T** Since aldosterone stimulates hydrogen and potassium secretion (as well as sodium reabsorption), excess aldosterone secretion can cause hydrogen ion loss and hence metabolic alkalosis — especially when plasma potassium is low **19.41**

(e) **T** Prolonged hypokalaemia causes loss of renal responsiveness to antidiuretic hormone **19.41, 19.35**

A332 (a) **F** This property is only possessed by the glucocorticoids and is due to stabilization of mast cell granules, decreased tissue synthesis of histamine and reduced formation of prostaglandins and kinins (due to stabilization of lysosomal membranes) **13.17**

(b) **F** There is an important contribution from suppression of the vascular response also **13.17**

(c) **T** By inhibiting extraneuronal uptake of noradrenaline they enhance vasoconstrictor influences and thereby contribute to the anti-inflammatory action **13.17**

(d) **F** The doses required to produce this effect are considerably higher than those that occur naturally **19.36**

(e) **T** Histamine release from mast cells is reduced due to stabilization of the granules, and histamine synthesis by the tissues is also suppressed **13.17**

A333 (a) **F** Embryologically the islets arise from the ducts associated with the gut and hepatic diverticula **19.43**

(b) **T** Thus the hepatocytes are exposed to higher levels of insulin and glucagon than are seen in the systemic circulation **19.43**

(c) **F** The β-cells do store insulin but they normally comprise 60–90% of the total number of islet cells **19.43**

(d) **F** All the β-cells secrete insulin; α-cells secrete glucagon, D-cells secrete somatostatin **19.43**

(e) **T** Unlike the acinar cells (which form the exocrine portion of the pancreas), the islets do not degenerate when the main pancreatic duct is ligated **19.43**

Q334 Insulin:

(a) is a large protein with a molecular weight of 30 000
(b) has a half-life of several hours in plasma
(c) is entirely degraded by the liver
(d) forms an insoluble complex with zinc in the pancreatic β-cells
(e) is normally secreted at a rate of about 50 U per day

Q335 In the fed state, increased insulin secretion:

(a) facilitates glucose transport in the intestinal mucosa
(b) suppresses hepatic glycogenolysis
(c) stimulates gluconeogenesis in the liver
(d) promotes amino acid uptake and protein synthesis in skeletal muscle
(e) reduces triglyceride synthesis in adipose tissue

Q336 In the fasting state, reduced insulin secretion:

(a) permits enhanced hepatic glycogenolysis to maintain blood glucose concentration
(b) prevents triglyceride breakdown
(c) acts synergistically with increased glucocorticoids to reduce skeletal muscle glucose uptake
(d) permits ketogenesis to occur in the liver
(e) may cause hypokalaemia

A334 (a) **F** Insulin consists of two peptide chains, one of 21 (A chain)   **19.44**
and one of 30 (B chain) residues. It is thus a small molecule with a molecular weight of 5700

(b) **F** The half-life of insulin is only a few minutes but its   **19.45**
maximal biological effects occur over 2–4 h since it binds to tissues

(c) **F** The liver removes 20–50% of insulin from the blood but   **19.45**
the pancreas and kidney (and placenta) are also involved in its degradation

(d) **T** The storage form of insulin consists of closely packed   **19.45**
arrays of zinc-insulin crystals

(e) **T** The average amount of insulin in the pancreas is 200 U   **19.45**
and the circulating (fasting) concentration is about 20 μU/ml

A335 (a) **F** Insulin increases glucose uptake in muscle, adipose   **19.46**
tissue, leucocytes, fibroblasts, the pituitary gland and liver but *not* in the intestine, kidney, brain or erythrocytes

(b) **T** By preventing the activation of glycogen phosphorylase,   **2.19,**
insulin acts to maintain glycogen stores   **19.46**

(c) **F** Insulin inhibits the liver enzymes involved in gluconeo-   **2.33,**
genesis; this action together with suppression of gly-   **19.46**
cogenolysis reduces glucose release into the blood

(d) **T** The amino acid uptake is dependent on concomitant   **19.46**
sodium uptake and the effects on protein metabolism act synergistically with those of growth hormone

(e) **F** Increased glucose uptake into adipocytes provides more   **19.46**
substrate for triglyceride synthesis

A336 (a) **T** However, this only lasts for a few hours — thereafter   **19.48**
increased gluconeogenesis (mainly in the liver) is respon- sible for maintaining fasting blood glucose levels

(b) **F** Insulin depresses lipolysis by inhibiting a lipase located   **19.47**
in adipocytes; reduced insulin thus permits accelerated triglyceride breakdown

(c) **T** Glucocorticoids are amongst several hormones released   **19.48**
when blood glucose levels fall

(d) **T** Increased free fatty acids, as a result of increased   **19.47**
lipolysis, are converted to ketone bodies in the liver and subsequently utilized by the central nervous system

(e) **F** Insulin promotes potassium uptake into cells; in its   **19.46**
absence, therefore, a reduction of plasma potassium would not be expected

Q337 Insulin release:

(a) is stimulated more effectively by intravenous than by oral administration of glucose

(b) is stimulated more effectively by glucagon when plasma glucose levels are high

(c) is stimulated by growth hormone

(d) is inhibited by vagal stimulation

(e) is under negative feedback control

Q338 Glucagon release is:

(a) stimulated by oral ingestion of glucose

(b) stimulated by intravenous infusion of glucose

(c) inhibited by atropine

(d) stimulated by muscular exercise

(e) stimulated by insulin

Q339 The relative molar concentrations of insulin and glucagon (I:G ratio):

(a) in a normal fasted subject is approximately 4

(b) rises after exhaustive exercise

(c) rises after glucose infusion

(d) rises after ingestion of a protein meal, providing that carbohydrate intake is adequate

(e) when high, is associated with lipolysis

A337 (a) **F** Despite achieving lower blood glucose concentrations, oral ingestion is the more effective stimulus since it also stimulates release of gastrointestinal hormones which potentiate the insulin-releasing action of nutrients and, themselves, stimulate insulin release   **19.49**

     (b) **T** Although evidence indicates that glucose and glucagon stimulate insulin release by different mechanisms or from different stored pools, their effects are synergistic   **19.49**

     (c) **F** Growth hormone stimulates the *synthesis* of insulin but does not directly influence release   **19.49**

     (d) **F** The cholinergic innervation of the islets is stimulatory whereas the noradrenergic innervation is inhibitory   **19.50**

     (e) **T** Apart from the effects of glucose, glucagon, and neurotransmitters on insulin release, insulin acts to reduce its own release from β-cells   **19.50**

A338 (a) **T** This response is probably mediated by cholecystokinin from the gut. The glucagon then acts on the β-cells to stimulate insulin release which inhibits further glucagon release   **19.62**

     (b) **F** Intravenous glucose administration depresses glucagon release, probably due to the inhibitory effect of insulin (released in response to the rise in blood glucose)   **19.62**

     (c) **T** The cholinergic innervation of the α_2-cells stimulates glucagon release; atropine lowers resting blood glucagon concentration   **19.62**

     (d) **T** This is probably due to increased noradrenergic efferent activity in the splanchnic nerve causing β-adrenoceptor-mediated secretion of glucagon   **19.61, 19.62**

     (e) **F** Insulin inhibits glucagon release, possibly due to a direct effect on α_2-cells or by increasing intracellular glucose levels in the α_2-cells   **19.61**

A339 (a) **T** It is thought this ratio is a better index of the interactive functioning of these hormones than are their plasma concentrations. The ratio can be as low as 0.4 in starvation or greater than 16 after glucose infusion   **19.62**

     (b) **F** It may fall to 0.4, thus facilitating glycogenolysis and gluconeogenesis and mobilizing endogenous fuel   **19.62**

     (c) **T** The rise (which can be up to 70) is largely due to increased insulin secretion with only a modest decline in glucagon   **19.63**

     (d) **T** With insufficient carbohydrate, the ratio falls because of decreased insulin release with reciprocal, increased glucagon   **19.63**

     (e) **F** Because of the action of insulin on lipase, a high I:G ratio is associated with inhibition of lipolysis   **19.63, 19.47**

Q340   In untreated diabetes mellitus:

(a)   fasting blood glucose concentration may be high
(b)   an increased urinary glucose concentration is due to the failure of insulin to promote glucose reabsorption in the kidney
(c)   reduced pyruvate production may lead to keto-acidosis
(d)   the plasma may have a milky appearance
(e)   an oral glucose load does not increase plasma insulin levels

Q341   Preparations used in insulin replacement therapy:

(a)   can be injected intravenously or subcutaneously
(b)   vary in the latency of onset of their action depending on the amount of zinc present
(c)   have a longer duration of action if they contain protein
(d)   may precipitate allergic reactions
(e)   contain the same amino acid sequence as human insulin

Q342   In the class of drugs used as oral hypoglycaemic agents:

(a)   the sulphonylureas act by stimulating insulin release
(b)   the biguanides act by stimulating glycolysis and reducing gluconeogenesis
(c)   tolbutamide is contraindicated in patients with renal insufficiency
(d)   chlorpropamide is contraindicated in patients with liver disease
(e)   phenformin may cause weight loss

A340 (a) **T** Due to a relative or absolute deficiency in insulin activity, blood glucose rises as a result of increased hepatic glycogenolysis and gluconeogenesis   **19.50**

(b) **F** The glycosuria is due to the fact that the amount of glucose filtered exceeds the maximum renal tubular reabsorptive capacity for glucose; insulin does not directly influence renal glucose transport   **19.46, 19.51**

(c) **T** A deficiency in the tricarboxylic acid cycle results in acetylcoenzyme A being diverted towards the production of ketone bodies   **19.51, 2.33**

(d) **T** This is due to the increased lipolysis, with the resulting elevation in free fatty acid levels   **19.51**

(e) **F** In some cases of maturity onset diabetes there is an exaggerated insulin response to glucose   **19.51, 19.52**

A341 (a) **F** All preparations must be injected, but several cannot be given intravenously because brisk hypoglycaemia would result   **19.55**

(b) **F** The presence of zinc increases the stability of the preparation and hence prolongs the duration of action, but the latency is affected by the amount of soluble insulin not complexed by protamine   **19.54**

(c) **T** Protamine or globin are used in some suspensions and, together with added zinc, produce a preparation of slow onset and long action   **19.54**

(d) **T** The protein in the preparation may stimulate an antigenic response, and the foreign insulin may induce antibody formation   **19.54, 19.56**

(e) **F** Pork insulin differs from human insulin by 1 amino acid, beef insulin by 3 amino acids   **19.54**

A342 (a) **T** For this reason they are rarely useful in juvenile diabetes where there is very little functional islet tissue   **19.57**

(b) **T** They also enhance glucose uptake into muscle in diabetic patients and thereby lower blood glucose   **19.60**

(c) **F** Tolbutamide is metabolized to an inactive form in the liver and is therefore contraindicated in patients with liver disease   **19.57**

(d) **F** Chlorpropamide is excreted unchanged in the urine, and is therefore contraindicated in renal insufficiency   **19.57, 19.58**

(e) **T** This is a common effect of the biguanides — probably attributable to the anorexia, nausea, vomiting and diarrhoea they cause   **19.60**

Q343 In normal man, plasma calcium concentration:

    (a)   lies between 60–70 mmol/l

    (b)   is lowered by the action of parathyroid hormone

    (c)   governs the release of calcitonin

    (d)   influences the membrane threshold potential in skeletal muscle and nerve

    (e)   regulates the formation of 25-hydroxycholecalciferol in the kidney

Q344 Parathyroid hormone:

    (a)   secretion is controlled by the anterior pituitary

    (b)   promotes the release of calcium and phosphate from bone

    (c)   promotes renal tubular calcium reabsorption

    (d)   is stored in the parathyroid glands

    (e)   inhibits the production of 1,25–dihydroxycholecalciferol in the kidney

Q345 Vitamin D:

    (a)   in the body is obtained from the diet

    (b)   is converted to active metabolites in the liver and kidney

    (c)   plays a permissive role in the action of parathyroid hormone

    (d)   facilitates the active absorption of calcium through the intestinal cell luminal membrane

    (e)   inhibits renal calcium reabsorption

A343 (a) F Normal plasma calcium concentration is about 2–2.5 mmol/l **19.64**

(b) F Parathyroid hormone acts synergistically with vitamin D to raise the plasma calcium concentration **19.64**

(c) T Calcitonin is released from the parafollicular cells of the thyroid in response to a rise in plasma calcium **19.68**

(d) T A change in the binding of calcium in the plasma membrane determines the potential at which the sodium channels open **5.13, 19.68**

(e) F 25–hydroxycholecalciferol is produced in the liver; it is metabolized to 1,25-dihydroxycholecalciferol in the kidney **19.66**

A344 (a) F Parathyroid hormone secretion occurs directly in response to changes in the ionized calcium concentration in plasma **19.65**

(b) T Due to an increase in the number of osteoclasts and increase in lysosomal enzyme, the bone matrix is broken down **19.68**

(c) T The action depends on stimulation of adenylate cyclase and production of cyclic AMP **19.68**

(d) F The glands contain no preformed hormone; parathyroid hormone is normally synthesized and secreted continuously **19.65**

(e) F There is some disagreement regarding the effects of parathyroid hormone on the metabolism of vitamin D, but it is either by increasing the production of the active 1,25-dihydroxycholecalciferol or through increased production of inactive 21,25–dihydroxycholecalciferol **19.67**

A345 (a) F Vitamin D is formed from steroid precursors in the skin in the presence of sunlight **43.8**

(b) T The liver converts vitamin D_3 to 25-hydroxycholecalciferol which is then converted to 1, 25-dihydroxycholecalciferol in the kidney **19.66**

(c) T The active metabolites of vitamin D stimulate the synthesis of calcium carrier proteins which mediate the transport of calcium into and out of bone cells **19.67, 19.68**

(d) T In response to a fall in plasma calcium, vitamin D is converted to its most active metabolite (1,25-dihydroxycholecalciferol) which then mediates intestinal calcium reabsorption via production of the carrier protein **19.67**

(e) F By stimulating synthesis of the calcium carrier protein, vitamin D enhances tubular reabsorption **19.68**

Q346 In man, calcitonin:

    (a)   is released from the parathyroid gland

    (b)   release is stimulated by a fall in the plasma calcium concentration

    (c)   principally acts on bone to suppress resorption and calcium release

    (d)   may be used in the treatment of vitamin D poisoning

    (e)   inhibits calcium absorption in the intestine

A346 (a) **F** Calcitonin is synthesized and released from the para-follicular cells of the thyroid   **19.68**

(b) **F** The stimulus for calcitonin secretion is a rise in plasma calcium   **19.69**

(c) **T** This effect is the opposite to that of parathyroid hormone   **19.69**

(d) **T** The hypercalcaemia which results from vitamin D poisoning (due to calcium mobilization from bone) can be offset by calcitonin   **19.69, 19.70**

(e) **F** Calcitonin does not influence intestinal calcium transport   **19.69**

General and Biochemical Pharmacology

Q347 The following drugs exert their pharmacological effects primarily as a consequence of the formation of covalent bonds with receptor molecules in the biological target tissue:

(a) organophosphorus anticholinesterases
(b) atropine
(c) metal ion chelating agents
(d) β-haloalkylamine, α-adrenoceptor antagonists (e.g. phenoxybenzamine)
(e) general anaesthetics

Q348 The following drugs exert their pharmacological effects primarily as a consequence of inhibition of one or more enzymes in biological tissues:

(a) penicillins
(b) aspirin
(c) isoprenaline
(d) acetazolamide
(e) heparin

A347 (a) **T** Covalent bonds are formed with the esteratic site of the enzyme. These bonds are broken with difficulty by H^+ donors such as oximes. This type of anticholinesterase is, therefore, almost irreversible in its action   **39.6, 10.37**

(b) **F** Atropine is a competitive antagonist of cholinomimetic agonists at muscarinic receptors. The atropine-receptor bond is almost certainly electrostatic; covalent bond formation would preclude competition by the agonist (see (a))   **39.6**

(c) **F** These form electrostatic bonds with di- or mono-valent metal ions   **39.9**

(d) **T** These agents are non-competitive antagonists since the covalent bonding reduces the number of receptors available to the agonist in an unsurmountable manner   **39.6, 11.41, 39.54**

(e) **F** These agents are possibly incorporated in clathrates by forming hydrophobic bonds with cell membrane components   **39.8**

A348 (a) **T** Penicillins inhibit the transpeptidases in bacteria   **39.12, 34.27**

(b) **T** Aspirin inhibits prostaglandin synthetases in a variety of tissues   **39.12, 12.33, 16.21**

(c) **F** Isoprenaline stimulates β-adrenoceptors which may secondarily involve activation of the enzyme adenylate cyclase   **11.32**

(d) **T** Acetazolamide inhibits carbonic anhydrase in the nephron, causing reduced bicarbonate reabsorption, increased bicarbonate excretion and diuresis   **39.12, 27.30**

(e) **T** Heparin, in combination with antithrombin III, combines with the coagulating enzyme thrombin, preventing the latter from converting fibrinogen to fibrin monomer. Heparin also neutralizes several clotting factors, but the anticoagulant effect is heavily dependent on thrombin inhibition   **39.12, 21.15**

Q349 It may be assumed that association and dissociation of a drug and its receptor can be expressed as a mass action equation, thus:

$$\text{Drug} + \text{Receptor} \underset{k_2}{\overset{k_1}{\rightleftharpoons}} \text{Drug–receptor complex}$$

or

$$D + R \underset{k_2}{\overset{k_1}{\rightleftharpoons}} DR$$

where k_1 is the association rate constant and k_2 the dissociation rate constant. It follows that, at equilibrium:

(a) $k_1 [D] [R] = k_2 [DR]$
(b) the proportion of the receptor sites occupied by drug will be inversely related to $[D]$
(c) k_2/k_1 is inversely related to the affinity of the drug for the receptor
(d) the pharmacological response will be related directly to $[DR]$ at the ED_{50} for the drug
(e) the pharmacological response will be related directly to $[D]$ at the ED_{50} for the drug

Q350 The relation between pharmacological response (ordinate) and the log concentration of an agonist drug (abscissa):

(a) is normally sigmoid in shape
(b) is normally linear over the range 20% to 80% of the maximum response
(c) is shifted leftwards in a parallel fashion by a competitive antagonist
(d) exhibits a reduced slope in the presence of an irreversible antagonist
(e) would be shifted to the right progressively for a series of related agonists with increasing efficacy (acting on the same receptors)

A349 (a) **T** Thus association and dissociation proceed at equal rates, which is the criterion for establishment of equilibrium   **39.16**

(b) **F** Up to a point, as [D] increases, so [DR] will increase and [R] (i.e. the number of free receptors) will fall, therefore [DR] is directly related to [D]   **39.17**

(c) **T** The reciprocal of k_2/k_1 is usually called the affinity constant (K) which increases with increasing affinity (thus association is faster than dissociation)   **39.19**

(d) **T** This is the basis of the occupancy theory of drug action and is an assumption which is supported by the available experimental evidence   **39.21**

(e) **T** The ED_{50} lies on the linear portion of the dose/response curve, thus the magnitude of the response is proportional to the drug concentration   **39.20**

A350 (a) **T** This is demonstrable for most agonists   **39.19**

(b) **T** This is demonstrable for most agonists   **39.19**

(c) **F** In the presence of a competitive antagonist the log concentration/response plot is shifted to the *right* in a parallel manner   **39.23**

(d) **T** With increasing concentration, an irreversible antagonist reduces the number of receptors available to the agonist, hence the maximum response and the slope of the log concentration/response plot are reduced   **39.27**

(e) **F** As efficacy increases, the log concentration/response curve shifts to the left   **39.35**

Q351 According to the occupation (occupancy) theory of drug-receptor interaction:

(a) pharmacological response is proportional to the fraction of the total number of receptors which is occupied by the agonist

(b) the occupation of a receptor by an agonist facilitates occupation of other adjacent receptors

(c) an all-or-none stimulus is elicited by the combination of each receptor site with an agonist molecule

(d) when the response is maximal, all the receptors are occupied

(e) when the response is maximal, the agonist concentration is equal to the dissociation constant for the agonist-receptor complex

Q352 For an agonist drug:

(a) the value of K_D is given by the molar concentration which generates half the maximal response

(b) the pD_2 value is the negative log of the dissociation constant

(c) a pD_2 value of 5 would indicate it had twice the potency of another agonist (acting on the same receptors) with a pD_2 of 5.3

(d) the pD_2 value is a measure of affinity

(e) the slope of the linear part of the log concentration:response plot indicates the magnitude of the pD_2 value

A351 (a) **T** This statement forms the basis of the occupation theory **39.19**
as proposed by A.J. Clark

(b) **F** It is assumed that occupation of one receptor *does not* **39.19**
affect the tendency of others to be occupied

(c) **T** It is further assumed that these individual all-or-none **39.19**
stimuli summate to produce the overall response

(d) **T** This assumption follows directly from the first (see (a)) **39.19**

(e) **F** The occupancy theory assumes that the dissociation **39.19**
constant is equal to the drug concentration at the *half*
maximal response, since

$$E/E_{max} = [D]/[D] + K_D \text{ (see equation [39.7], p.\textbf{39.19})}$$
$$\text{if } \tfrac{1}{2} = [D]/[D] + K_D$$
$$\text{then } K_D = [D]$$

A352 (a) **T** K_D is the dissociation constant which is equal to the ED_{50} **39.20**
in molar units

(b) **T** This is the definition of pD_2 which gives a value for **34.19,**
potency of agonism **39.28**

(c) **F** A pD_2 of 5 would indicate an ED_{50} of 10^{-5} M whilst a pD_2 **39.19**
of 5.3 would indicate an ED_{50} of $10^{-5.3}$ (i.e. half of 10^{-5}
or 5×10^{-6} M). Thus a pD_2 of 5 would indicate *half* the
potency of a compound with a pD_2 of 5.3

(d) **T** The pD_2 is the most common measure of affinity in **39.19**
concentration:response terms

(e) **F** The members of an agonist series may produce different **39.28**
maximum responses and hence different slopes to the log
concentration:response plot, but they may have the same
or similar pD_2 values

Q353 For a given antagonist drug:

(a) the pA_2 value is the negative logarithm of the molar concentration which will reduce the potency of an agonist (acting on the same receptors) by half

(b) the pA_2 value is always less than the pA_{10}

(c) the difference between the pA_2 and the pA_{10} can be used to distinguish competitive from non-competitive (irreversible) antagonism

(d) a high pA_2 value indicates non-specific antagonism

(e) a pA_2 value of 7 would indicate that it had twice the potency of another antagonist (acting on the same receptors) with a pA_2 of 8

Q354 Drugs which may be described as partial agonists:

(a) cannot elicit the same maximum response, irrespective of concentration, as a pure agonist acting on the same receptors

(b) will, at certain concentrations, inhibit the effects of a pure agonist acting on the same receptors

(c) have an intrinsic activity which is greater than unity

(d) elicit a maximum response, in a given tissue, which is inversely related in magnitude to their intrinsic activity

(e) show an antagonist potency which is greater, the higher the affinity for the receptors

A353 (a) **T** This is the definition of the pA_2 value which represents, in a single value, the potency of an antagonist drug with respect to a particular agonist   **39.24**

(b) **F** The pA_{10} value is the negative logarithm of the antagonist concentration (molar units) which reduces the potency of an agonist to 0.1 of the original value. Hence the pA_{10} is always less than the pA_2 **39.24**

(c) **T** For competitive antagonists the pA_2 minus the pA_{10} lies between 0.8 and 1.2; a gross departure from this indicates non-competitive or irreversible antagonism   **39.24**

(d) **F** Low pA_2 values are obtained when antagonism is unspecific   **39.24**

(e) **F** A drug with a pA_2 of 7 would reduce the potency of an agonist by half at a concentration of 10^{-7}M (see (a)). A drug with a pA_2 of 8 would have the same effect at 10^{-8}M and hence would be ten times more potent   **39.24**

A354 (a) **T** By definition, a drug which does not elicit the maximum response from a tissue, even when all the receptors are occupied (occupancy theory) or stimulated at maximal frequency (rate theory), is a partial agonist   **39.27**

(b) **T** This antagonist property increases with concentration, thus at low concentrations the agonist property predominates and at the higher concentrations the drugs progressively exert their antagonistic effects   **39.27**

(c) **F** Intrinsic activity is a constant relating degree of receptor occupancy, or activation, to concentration. For a pure agonist intrinsic activity is 1, for a pure antagonist it is 0 and for partial agonists intrinsic activity lies between these values   **39.28**

(d) **F** As described above, the maximum response is related *directly*, though not necessarily linearly, to the intrinsic activity   **39.28, Fig. 39.17**

(e) **T** As affinity increases (and therefore the dissociation constant decreases) so the antagonist component of the action of partial agonists increases   **39.33**

Q355   According to the rate theory of drug action:

(a)   the stimulus provided by an agonist will be proportional to the rate of formation of agonist–receptor complexes

(b)   drugs which associate rapidly with receptors will tend to be potent agonists

(c)   drugs which dissociate rapidly from receptors will tend to be potent antagonists

(d)   the rate of formation of drug–receptor complexes will be maximal at the steepest point on the log concentration response plot

(e)   with increasing concentration, partial agonists will show progressively decreasing rates of dissociation from receptors

Q356   The development of tachyphylaxis (relatively brisk diminution of response to successive applications of the same dose of an agonist drug):

(a)   indicates that, at a higher dose, the drug must be a partial agonist

(b)   to an agonist is never associated with a decreased response to other agonists acting on the same tissue but via different receptors

(c)   to tyramine is due to α-adrenoceptor desensitization

(d)   is seen with suxamethonium at the motor end plate

(e)   to acetylcholine at the motor end plate causes desensitization that is restricted to drugs acting on the nicotinic receptor

A355 (a) **T** This is the basic assumption of the rate theory as proposed by Paton — **39.40**

(b) **F** The rate of association can be high for both agonists and antagonists — **39.40, 39.42**

(c) **F** The rate theory assumes that agonists dissociate rapidly and antagonists dissociate slowly — **39.40**

(d) **F** The rate theory assumes that the rate of formation of drug–receptor complexes is maximal at the maximum response — **39.40**

(e) **T** Hence antagonism increases with increasing concentration — **39.42**

A356 (a) **F** Tachyphylaxis may indicate partial agonism, but there are several other possible mechanisms (see (b)) — **39.52**

(b) **F** Receptor-specific tachyphylaxis is seen with 5-hydroxytryptamine on smooth muscle, but tachyphylaxis to acetylcholine usually provokes a decreased response to other agonists such as histamine. This may be due to loss of intracellular potassium ions — **39.52**

(c) **F** Tyramine acts by promoting release of noradrenaline from a limited pool in the noradrenergic nerve terminal. This pool is briskly depleted by successive doses of tyramine — **39.52**

(d) **T** Suxamethonium is a partial agonist, initially depolarizing and then blocking the receptors of the motor end plate — **39.58**

(e) **T** Acetylcholine tachyphylaxis extends to other nicotonic agonists but not to potassium ions or caffeine — **39.59**

Q357 Adrenoceptors:

(a) of the α type always mediate contraction in smooth muscle

(b) of the β type are resistant to blockade by phenoxybenzamine

(c) of the β type always mediate synthesis of cyclic AMP

(d) of the β type are not selective towards the optical isomers of adrenaline or noradrenaline

(e) of the β_1 type give a higher pD_2 value for isoprenaline than for noradrenaline

Q358 The passage of a drug across biological membranes:

(a) is rapid for molecules with a high oil/water partition coefficient

(b) is low for large, water-soluble molecules which are not ligands for transmembrane carrier systems

(c) is higher for ionized forms of the drug than for non-ionized forms

(d) is inversely related to the pK_a of the molecule

(e) is low for drugs that bind tightly to plasma proteins

Q359 Dissolution of a drug administered in tablet form:

(a) is increased by addition of sodium bicarbonate to the medium comprising the tablet

(b) is greater, the smaller the drug particle size

(c) is reduced by addition of surfactants to the tablet

(d) is reduced in the stomach by tablet coatings which are more soluble in alkali than in acid

(e) is usually greater for drugs in the crystalline form than in the amorphous form

A357 (a) **F** For many types of smooth muscle this is true, but in the intestine there are α-adrenoceptors which mediate relaxation of smooth muscle via an increase in potassium ion permeability   **39.65**

(b) **T** Phenoxybenzamine blocks α-adrenoceptors and histamine and 5-hydroxytryptamine receptors, but has little or no effect on β-adrenoceptors   **39.66, 39.54**

(c) **F** It is possible to generate positive inotropy in the myocardium via β-adrenoceptors without synthesis of cyclic AMP   **39.65**

(d) **F** For both agonists the (–) isomer is much more potent   **39.66**

(e) **T** Isoprenaline is a more potent β_1-adrenoceptor agonist than noradrenaline, hence its pD_2 value would be higher   **9.17**

A358 (a) **T** As lipid solubility increases (hence the oil/water partition coefficient increases) so the solubility in membrane lipids enables rapid passage   **40.2**

(b) **T** Large molecules which are water soluble have low oil/water partition coefficients; they cannot permeate pores, and cross membranes readily only if their chemical structure enables them to 'take advantage' of physiological carrier mechanisms   **40.2**

(c) **F** Ionization reduces lipid solubility and reduces membrane permeability. Ionization tends to cause hydration of the molecule in solution which also impairs lipid solubility   **40.3**

(d) **F** K_a is the ionization constant, so as K_a increases, ionization increases and membrane permeability falls. The pK_a is the negative logarithm of K_a (alternatively pK_a = $1/K_a$), thus as K_a rises, pK_a falls. So, as pK_a falls, membrane permeability falls   **40.3**

(e) **T** Binding to large molecules, which do not cross membranes readily, reduces the transfer of the bound drug   **40.6**

A359 (a) **T** On exposure to gastric acid the sodium bicarbonate forms carbon dioxide, the bubbles of which help to break up the tablet   **40.8**

(b) **T** The smaller the particle size, the larger the ratio of surface area to mass, and the more rapidly the drug dissolves in water   **40.9**

(c) **F** Surfactants reduce the surface tension and are sometimes added to tablets as excipients which *increase* the solubility of the drug   **40.9**

(d) **T** These are called enteric coatings and are used to protect the gastric lining against drugs which irritate it. The enteric coating is dissolved by the alkaline secretions of the small intestine in which the drug is absorbed   **40.8**

(e) **F** Where a difference exists, the amorphous form is the more soluble   **40.9**

Q360 Absorption from the gastrointestinal tract:

(a) may be higher in the stomach than in the small intestine for acidic drugs

(b) of tetracyclines may be impaired when taken with milk

(c) avoids passage of a drug through the liver before it enters the systemic circulation

(d) is likely to be higher for an acidic drug with a low pK_a than for a basic drug with a high pK_a

(e) may occur for certain drugs, by co-absorption with dietary lipids

Q361 Administration of a drug:

(a) by the sublingual route avoids first-pass inactivation in the liver

(b) in the form of rectal suppositories exposes the drug to first-pass hepatic inactivation

(c) by inhalation prevents systemic effects

(d) which is ionized may be achieved through the skin by electrophoresis

(e) which is irritant to tissues, would be unsafe if made intravenously

A360 (a) **F** Although acidic drugs are less ionized at low pH (e.g. in gastric acid) and the unionized form is more readily absorbed, more absorption occurs through the greater surface area of small intestine **40.11**

(b) **T** Tetracyclines form insoluble chelates with polyvalent metal ions; the calcium ions in milk are particularly effective in this respect **40.13**

(c) **F** The venous drainage from both stomach and intestine carries drugs directly to the liver via the hepatic portal circulation **40.14**

(d) **F** The acidic drug will be more readily absorbed in the stomach whilst the basic drug will be more readily absorbed in the small intestine. However, the surface area available for absorption in the small intestine is much greater than that offered by the stomach **40.12**

(e) **T** Drugs such as digoxin and griseofulvin, which are highly lipid soluble, are more readily absorbed when taken after a high fat meal. The drugs cross the membranes in combination with long-chain fatty acids, monoglycerides or fat-soluble vitamins **40.10**

A361 (a) **T** The drug enters systemic capillaries, returns to the right atrium and passes into the systemic circulation after passage through the lungs; the hepatic portal system is thus avoided **40.15**

(b) **T** Only a proportion of the rectal venous drainage enters the vena cava directly without entering the portal circulation **40.15**

(c) **F** Although inhalation may reduce systemic effects (as, for example, with β-adrenoceptor agonists in asthma) appreciable plasma levels may still be attained **40.16**

(d) **T** Methacholine (as a vasodilator) and certain local anaesthetics can be administered by driving the charged particles through the skin by electrophoresis **40.16**

(e) **F** Intravenous administration is an acceptable and sometimes preferable route for irritant drugs **40.17**

Q362 The distribution in the body of a drug:

    (a)   may be altered by acidosis

    (b)   may depend upon the obesity of the patient

    (c)   may be described by the volume of distribution (V_d), which is the volume of solution that would be formed if the total amount of drug in the body were dissolved at the plasma concentration

    (d)   is restricted for non-lipid-soluble anionic drugs because they bind to plasma albumin

    (e)   with a volume of distribution of about 0.2 l/kg would be confined to the vascular compartment

Q363 Binding of a drug to plasma albumin:

    (a)   may attenuate the pharmacological effect

    (b)   may increase the effects of another drug taken simultaneously

    (c)   may promote allergic reactions to the drug

    (d)   may reduce excretion of the drug via the kidneys

    (e)   is more extensive in neonates than in adults

A362 (a) **T** For drugs with a pK_a close to the pH of plasma, changes **40.18**
in the hydrogen ion concentration in blood will shift the
dissociation of the drug. Thus in acidosis an acidic drug
will be relatively less dissociated and achieve a wider
distribution

(b) **T** Thiopentone, for instance, is slowly taken up by fat cells; **40.18**
the more fat, the more thiopentone sequestered by it

(c) **T** This is the definition of the volume of distribution which **40.19**
serves as a single value for comparison of different
drugs

(d) **F** Lipid-soluble and/or cationic drugs bind preferentially to **40.20**
plasma albumin — the protein has a net anionic charge
(isoelectric point at pH 4.9) and hydrophobic side-chains
of amino acid residues

(e) **F** A drug confined to the plasma volume would have an **40.19**
apparent volume of distribution of about 0.6 l/kg. A value
of 0.2 l/kg would be observed for a drug that was distributed in the extracellular fluid

A363 (a) **T** Only the free molecules in solution exert a pharma- **40.23**
cological effect, thus binding of some fraction by plasma
albumin reduces the response

(b) **T** If both drugs tend to bind to plasma albumin, but one **40.24**
binds more effectively than the other, then the
pharmacological effects of the less bound drug will be
amplified

(c) **T** Small molecules which bind to the large protein **13.23**
molecules can alter the immunological identity of the
latter sufficiently to render them antigenic; such small
molecules are called haptens. Albumin is not the only
plasma protein involved in such reactions, but it has
been implicated in some cases

(d) **·T** Drug molecules bound tightly to albumin are not readily **40.30**
filtered through the glomerulus

(e) **F** Neonates are hypoalbuminaemic (low plasma albumin) **40.24**
and hence have a *reduced* drug binding capacity

Q364 Passage of drugs into:

(a) adipose tissue occurs rapidly if they are lipid-soluble
(b) the brain is restricted for drugs which are bound to plasma proteins
(c) the brain occurs readily for drugs which are highly ionized at plasma pH
(d) the fetal circulation depends upon the pK_a value
(e) the urine may occur by renal tubular secretion

Q365 With reference to excretion of drugs by the kidneys:

(a) no drugs enter the urine without some metabolic change to their structure
(b) certain drugs can increase plasma uric acid concentration by a renal mechanism
(c) acidification of the urine will reduce the excretion of basic drugs which normally undergo tubular re-absorption
(d) renal clearance is equal to the concentration of the drug in urine divided by its concentration in plasma
(e) a clearance ratio of greater than unity indicates that the drug has been secreted by the tubules

A364 (a) **F** Adipose tissue has a very low blood flow. Lipid-soluble drugs may be sequestered in large amounts in fat, but uptake is slow   **40.26**

(b) **T** The capillaries in the central nervous system have tight junctions between the endothelial cells forming the so-called blood–brain barrier; drugs bound to plasma proteins do not readily cross   **40.28**

(c) **F** The ionized form will not readily cross the membranes of the endothelial cells of the central nervous system capillaries (see (b))   **40.29**

(d) **T** The placenta has the general properties of a lipid membrane barrier which is crossed most readily by non-ionized lipid-soluble molecules   **20.41**

(e) **T** A wide range of drugs is secreted actively by the renal tubules   **40.31, Table 40.20**

A365 (a) **F** Acetazolamide, amiloride, aminocaproic acid, cromoglycate, frusemide and pentolinium are all excreted unchanged by the kidneys   **40.31**

(b) **T** Thiazide diuretics, salicylates, phenylbutazone and probenecid compete with uric acid for secretion into the tubular fluid leading to hyperuricaemia and possibly gout   **40.31**

(c) **F** In more acid urine, basic drugs are more ionized; the ionic form will be reabsorbed less rapidly and excretion will be increased   **40.32**

(d) **F** Renal clearance relates the *amount* of drug excreted in the urine to the plasma concentration, hence renal clearance = urine concentration × rate of urine formation/plasma concentration   **40.33**

(e) **T** The clearance ratio relates drug clearance to inulin clearance or glomerular filtration rate. Inulin is not secreted or reabsorbed, hence the only way a clearance ratio of greater than unity can occur is through the secretion of the drug into tubular fluid   **40.33**

Q366 Oxidative metabolic reactions involving drugs:

- (a) are examples of Phase II metabolism
- (b) may be catalysed by hepatic microsomal enzyme systems
- (c) include deamination
- (d) may occur in mitochondria
- (e) may occur in noradrenaline storage vesicles

Q367 In drug metabolism, phase I reactions:

- (a) lead to the production of compounds with little or no pharmacological activity
- (b) of the reduction type do not occur in hepatic microsomal enzymes
- (c) include amide hydrolysis
- (d) include hydrolysis of ester groups which occurs only in the liver
- (e) must occur before conjugative reactions are possible

A366 (a) **F** Oxidative reactions are Phase I; Phase II reactions are conjugative — 40.35

(b) **T** These reactions frequently occur in the liver and may be mimicked *in vitro* using hepatic microsomal subcellular fractions — 40.35

(c) **T** Deamination can be oxidative, for example for amphetamine the primary amine group is oxidized to -NHOH to yield hydroxylamine — 40.36, 26.19

(d) **T** The mitochondrial enzyme monoamine oxidase deaminates (oxidatively) catecholamines, sympathomimetic amines, 5-hydroxytryptamine and N-methylhistamine — 40.36, 11.6

(e) **T** Dopamine-β-hydroxylase is present in noradrenaline storage vesicles; it catalyses oxidative hydroxylation of dopamine to noradrenaline and participates in the synthesis of false transmitter substances such as α-methyl noradrenaline (from α-methyl dopa via α-methyl dopamine) — 40.36, 11.3

A367 (a) **F** Phase I reactions can produce compounds with significant or even enhanced pharmacological activity (c.f. phenacetin conversion to paracetamol); these are called active metabolites — 40.35

(b) **F** Hepatic microsomal enzymes can reduce azo- and nitrogroups to the corresponding amine groups, and can catalyse reductive dehalogenation as, for example, in the conversion of halothane to trifluoroethane — 40.37

(c) **T** Amide hydrolysis is relatively slow, hence procainamide is more slowly excreted than procaine, thereby lengthening its antiarrhythmic effect — 40.37

(d) **F** Esterases are widely distributed; for instance, many drugs are acted upon by plasma esterases — 40.37

(e) **F** Some drugs are directly conjugated; nicotinamide, chloramphenicol, paracetamol, morphine are a few examples — 40.38

Q368 In drug metabolism, phase II reactions:

    (a)   include hepatic glucuronide conjugation

    (b)   may produce toxic metabolites

    (c)   may be saturated by clinical doses of certain drugs

    (d)   generally produce compounds which are substantially ionized at plasma pH

    (e)   may involve acetyl coenzyme A

A368 (a) **T** Many drugs are conjugated with UDP-glucuronic acid; **40.38**
this occurs in the hepatocyte

(b) **T** Conjugative reactions rarely produce toxic metabolites, **40.43**
but certain conjugates have low urine solubility, crystal-
lizing out in the tubules and damaging the kidney

(c) **T** For aspirin, doses in excess of 1 g saturate glucuronide **40.39**
conjugation and the proportion of unchanged salicylic
acid excreted increases

(d) **F** As **Table 40.28** shows, conjugation involves hydroxyl, **40.39**
sulphydryl or amine groups. Since these groups are
those that normally ionize, the conjugates are less
ionized than the parent drug and are therefore more
readily secreted

(e) **T** In the formation of acetyl conjugates, the acetyl group is **40.38**
transferred from acetyl coenzyme A

Medical Microbiology and Chemotherapy

Q369 Among antimicrobial drugs:

(a) sulphonamides act by inhibiting essential metabolic reactions confined to the microorganism

(b) cephalosporins interfere with the synthesis of the bacterial cell wall

(c) penicillins disorientate the structure of the plasma membrane inside the bacterial cell wall

(d) the aminoglycosides act on bacterial ribosomes to impair protein synthesis

(e) chloramphenicol acts on bacterial DNA to prevent replication

Q370 With reference to antimicrobial drugs:

(a) the tetracyclines are primarily bactericidal

(b) chloramphenicol has a broad spectrum of activity

(c) the polymyxins act mainly against Gram-positive organisms

(d) the cephalosporins act mainly against Gram-positive organisms

(e) certain antibiotics free non-susceptible bacteria from competition by susceptible bacteria

A369 (a) **T** Hence the microorganism is affected and the host unaffected   **34.16**

     (b) **T** Host cells do not have cell walls, hence the drug, by inhibiting cell wall synthesis, causes the bacteria to rupture in a hypotonic environment   **34.16**

     (c) **F** Penicillins act like cephalosporins (see (a)); polymyxin and thyrothrycin disorientate bacterial plasma membranes without binding to those of the host cells   **34.16**

     (d) **T** These drugs do not affect protein-synthesis in the host cells either because they do not enter the cells or do not bind to the ribosomal enzymes   **34.16**

     (e) **F** No known drugs act this way; chloramphenicol acts in the same manner as the aminoglycosides (see (d))   **34.16**

A370 (a) **F** Tetracyclines are primarily bacteriostatic, that is they prevent growth and multiplication of bacteria without killing the mature organisms   **34.17**

     (b) **T** It acts on a range of Gram-positive and Gram-negative bacteria   **34.18**

     (c) **F** The polymyxins act mainly against Gram-negative organisms   **34.18**

     (d) **T** This may be demonstrated using selective bacterial cultures   **34.18**

     (e) **T** This is called superinfection and is commonly seen when bacteria which suppress staphylococci or *Candida albicans* are killed by antibiotics   **34.19**

Q371 Sulphonamides:

    (a)   are more effective than penicillins in the treatment of lobar pneumonia

    (b)   inhibit folic acid synthesis in certain types of bacteria

    (c)   are particularly effective against purulent infections

    (d)   may be used for local infections of the eye, ear and nose

    (e)   of the less soluble varieties may form crystals in the urine

Q372 Inhibition of the synthesis of folic acid:

    (a)   is a property of p-aminobenzoic acid

    (b)   is a property of trimethoprim

    (c)   in *Mycobacterium leprae* is the mechanism of action of the sulphones against leprosy

    (d)   leads to impairment of synthesis of nucleic acids in certain bacteria

    (e)   in mammalian cells accounts for some of the side-effects of certain antibiotics

A371 (a) **F** Lobar pneumonia is caused by *Streptococcus pneumo-*   **34.24**
      niae and, although sulphonamides are effective against
      this organism, penicillins are more so and, currently, are
      the treatment of choice

    (b) **T** The sulphonamides are structural analogues of p-   **34.20**
      aminobenzoic acid, which is part of the folic acid
      molecule. Folic acid is essential for DNA and RNA syn-
      thesis and since certain bacteria cannot take up folate
      from the surrounding medium, they must synthesize it.
      Thus, the inhibition of folate synthesis by sulphonamides
      impedes nucleic acid synthesis in these bacteria

    (c) **F** The pus produced in purulent infections contains the   **34.20**
      end-products of cell breakdown, including the raw
      materials for folic acid synthesis. The presence of pus,
      therefore, reduces the efficacy of sulphonamides

    (d) **T** The sulphonamides sulphacetamide, sulphafurazole die-   **34.20**
      thanolamine and mafenide are non-irritant and are
      widely used by topical administration for infections of
      this type

    (e) **T** Crystalluria and diarrhoea are the most serious of the   **34.24**
      side-effects of sulphonamides. These are indications for
      immediate withdrawal of the drug because crystalluria
      can lead to renal tubular blockage, anuria and tubular
      necrosis

A372 (a) **F** p-Aminobenzoic acid is one of the precursors of folic acid   **34.20**
      and is therefore used in its synthesis

    (b) **T** Trimethoprim is a relatively weak inhibitor of dihydro-   **34.24**
      folate reductase, but this is the mechanism of its
      bacteriostatic action

    (c) **T** The sulphones are the most important antibiotics in the   **34.25**
      treatment of leprosy. They act by inhibition of folic acid
      synthesis in *Myco. leprae*

    (d) **T** Certain bacteria cannot take up folic acid and must,   **34.20**
      therefore, synthesize it since it is a component of their
      DNA and RNA

    (e) **F** Mammalian cells can take up folic acid from extra-   **34.20**
      cellular fluid and can therefore synthesize DNA and
      RNA in the presence of inhibitors of folic acid synthesis.
      (Folic acid is, however, a vital component of the
      mammalian diet)

Q373 Benzylpenicillin:

(a) is almost totally absorbed from the stomach after oral administration
(b) has a renal clearance value which is equal to the glomerular filtration rate
(c) is active only against Gram-negative organisms
(d) is active against *Streptococci*
(e) inhibits the formation of peptide cross-linkages essential for bacterial cell wall synthesis

Q374 Penicillins:

(a) are relatively toxic drugs with a wide range of side-effects
(b) promote antibody synthesis in about 5–10% of patients
(c) induce, in some bacteria, penicillinase enzymes that enable these organisms to resist the antibiotic effect
(d) of the partially synthetic varieties may be resistant to penicillinases
(e) of the partially synthetic varieties may be more resistant to gastric acid than is benzylpenicillin

Q375 The following antibiotics act by inhibiting bacterial cell wall synthesis:

(a) cephalosporins
(b) cephamycins
(c) aminoglycosides
(d) polymyxins
(e) rifamycins

A373 (a) F   Benzylpenicillin is rapidly destroyed by acidic gastric   **34.28**
juice and under the most favourable conditions only
about 30% of an oral dose is absorbed. Most of this
absorption occurs from the small intestine

(b) F   This would imply that benzylpenicillin was filtered but   **34.28**
neither secreted nor reabsorbed by the tubule. In fact,
tubular secretion occurs because benzylpenicillin binds
to the secretory carrier for weak acids

(c) F   The penicillins act against *Neisseria* which is Gram-   **34.27**
negative, but they also act against a range of Gram-
positive organisms

(d) T'   These include pneumococci; the penicillins also act   **34.27**
against other Gram-positive organisms such as
*Staphylococci, Corynebacteria, Bacilli, Clostridia,
Actinomyces* and *Treponema*

(e) T   This is the major mode of action which occurs through   **34.27**
inhibition of a transpeptidase enzyme

A374 (a) F   Penicillins are the least toxic of the antibiotics, side-   **34.30**
effects are few and are largely restricted to allergic
reactions

(b) F   Antibody synthesis occurs in *all* patients, but the   **34.30**
presence of these antibodies generates allergic
reactions in only 5–10% of patients

(c) T   This is the usual basis of bacterial resistance to the   **34.28**
penicillins. The penicillinases hydrolyse the penicillin to
inactive penicillinoic acids

(d) T   The acquisition of this property has been one of the   **34.31,**
major successes of the semi-synthetic penicillins,   **Table**
although resistance to the enzyme is never total   **34.7**

(e) T   Many of the semi-synthetic penicillins are resistant to   **34.31,**
destruction by gastric acid and are therefore more effec-   **Table**
tively absorbed after oral administration   **34.7**

A375 (a) T   The cephalosporins act in the same way as the   **34.34**
penicillins but are resistant to penicillinase enzymes in
bacteria

(b) T   These are active against some bacteria which are   **34.36**
resistant to other cell wall synthesis inhibitors, but they
are inactive orally and must be injected

(c) F   The aminoglycosides act on bacterial ribosomes to   **34.37**
impair protein synthesis

(d) F   The polymyxins bind to the plasma membranes of   **34.38**
certain bacteria causing a leakage of small molecules
such as phosphates and nucleosides. The loss of these
substances reduces the survival of the bacteria

(e) F   These inhibit bacterial synthesis of ribonucleic acids,   **34.38**
impairing protein synthesis

Medical Microbiology and Chemotherapy   345

Q376 Streptomycin:

(a) induces enzymes in bacteria, leading to resistance to its effects

(b) is well absorbed from the gastrointestinal tract

(c) crosses the blood–brain barrier when the meninges are inflamed

(d) inhibits bacterial protein synthesis by acting on certain ribosomal subunits

(e) may have toxic effects on the eighth cranial nerve

Q377 The tetracyclines:

(a) bind to bacterial ribosomes and impede protein synthesis

(b) have a narrow spectrum of activity, acting only against a small range of Gram-positive organisms

(c) are predominantly bactericidal

(d) are accumulated by sensitive, but not by resistant, strains of bacteria

(e) are accumulated in the teeth of children, causing hypoplasia of dental enamel

Q378 Chloramphenicol:

(a) impairs bacterial protein synthesis by inhibiting the elongation of peptide chains

(b) is toxic to bone marrow and can cause aplastic anaemia

(c) acts on bacteria in a similar manner to erythromycin

(d) is restricted in its use to the treatment of typhoid and paratyphoid fevers

(e) does not cause resistance to develop in susceptible bacteria

A376	(a)	F	Resistance to streptomycin is acquired by strains of bacteria due to the development of resistant mutants	34.40
	(b)	F	Most of an oral dose is excreted in the faeces and thus it is usually given by intramuscular injection	34.40
	(c)	T	The inflammation of tuberculous meningitis increases the permeability of the cerebral capillaries thereby admitting the drug to the cerebrospinal fluid. It was the first antibiotic to be effective in this disease	34.40
	(d)	T	Streptomycin acts on 30s ribosomal subunits, the smaller subunit of the ribosome which binds messenger RNA	34.40
	(e)	T	This is unexplained, but is the most serious side-effect, leading to vertigo, tinnitus and sometimes deafness	34.40

A377	(a)	T	They bind to the 30s subunit of the ribosomes and interfere with the binding of messenger RNA. They also bind to the messenger RNA itself; both actions impede protein synthesis	34.41
	(b)	F	They are broad-spectrum antibiotics acting against a range of both Gram-positive and Gram-negative bacteria	34.41
	(c)	F	They are bacteriostatic, impeding growth and multiplication rather than killing the bacteria	34.41
	(d)	T	They pass into sensitive bacteria more readily than they leave. Resistant strains tend not to accumulate tetracyclines, since they pass into and out of the bacterial cells equally readily	34.41
	(e)	T	Because they chelate divalent metal ions, especially calcium, they accumulate in growing teeth and bones and can suppress enamel formation. This effect may be manifest as discolouration of the teeth	34.42

A378	(a)	T	It binds to the larger (50s) ribosomes of bacteria and prevents the movement of these ribosomes along messenger RNA	34.43
	(b)	T	The mechanism of this effect is unknown, but its seriousness restricts the use of the drug	34.43
	(c)	T	Erythromycin also binds to 50s ribosomes in bacteria (see (a))	34.44
	(d)	T	It is the drug of choice for these serious infections and, although it acts on many other bacteria, its bone marrow suppressant effects preclude its use in other conditions	34.43
	(e)	F	There are various mechanisms responsible for the development of resistance in strains of bacteria which are susceptible prior to treatment	34.43

Q379 The antifungal drug, griseofulvin:

(a) is effective against ringworm caused by all known forms of fungi

(b) is used by topical administration and may not be given orally

(c) is normally used in combination with topical zinc undecenoate or tolnaftate

(d) can inhibit mammalian cell division

(e) has a broader spectrum of action than clotrimazole

Q380 Nystatin:

(a) is used in the treatment of candidiasis

(b) binds selectively to biological membranes which do not contain sterols

(c) does not exert toxic effects on mammalian cells

(d) acts on fungi in a manner which differs from that of amphotericin

(e) is the drug of choice for the treatment of pulmonary aspergillosis

A379 (a) **T** Griseofulvin is active against all ringworm (tinea) infec- **35.4,**
tions due to both the associated genera of fungi (*Tricho-* **Table**
phyton and *Microsporum*) **35.1**

(b) **F** Griseofulvin is inactive topically when used in conven- **35.5**
tional ointment bases; currently it is always given orally

(c) **T** Oral griseofulvin in combination with these topical anti- **35.5**
fungals is the therapy of choice for dermatomycoses
(fungal infections of the skin)

(d) **T** This occurs at concentrations which are greater than **35.5**
those achieved in clinical use. Griseofulvin depoly-
merizes microtubules thereby preventing formation of
the mitotic spindle and arresting cell division in
metaphase

(e) **F** Griseofulvin is predominantly active against fungi **35.6**
causing tinea infections. Clotrimazole (and miconazole)
are active not only against tinea but also against *Candida*
and other types of fungi

A380 (a) **T** Nystatin is used both topically and orally for the **35.7**
treatment of all forms of *Candida* infection

(b) **F** Nystatin does not bind to sterol-free membranes such as **35.7**
those found in bacteria, hence the drug is not toxic to
bacteria. Membranes of fungi and protozoa, which
contain sterols, bind nystatin and this renders these
organisms susceptible

(c) **F** Mammalian cell membranes contain sterols (see (b)) and **35.7**
are affected by nystatin. The toxic effects of the drug are
restricted because there is some selectivity towards
fungi and because absorption is poor from either topical
or oral administration

(d) **F** Amphotericin and nystatin both bind to sterol-containing **35.8**
membranes and impair the maintenance of a normal
intracellular environment in fungi

(e) **F** Pulmonary aspergillosis has been treated with nystatin **35.9**
but the most effective and reliable method of treatment
is prolonged systemic amphotericin

Q381 The malarial parasite (*Plasmodium*):

(a) reproduces sexually in the mammalian host but not in the mosquito

(b) first enters erythrocytes and later hepatocytes in a freshly infected mammal

(c) produces pyrogens when affected erythrocytes burst causing episodic fever

(d) may result in a dark colouration of the urine

(e) is not acutely lethal in some individuals

Q382 The antimalarial drug(s):

(a) are active only against the erythrocytic stages of the parasite

(b) quinine is sequestered by erythrocytes infected with *Plasmodium*

(c) chloroquine inhibits plasmodial nucleic acid synthesis

(d) chloroquine is more toxic to man than is quinine

(e) can be used prophylactically

A381 (a) **F** Sexual reproduction, between male microgametes and female macrogametes, occurs in the stomach of the mosquito producing sporozoites which can infect mammals bitten by the mosquito **36.5**

(b) **F** On entering the bloodstream of a new mammalian host the sporozoites enter hepatocytes where the exoerythrocytic stages of reproduction occur. Erythrocytes are affected 5–15 days later **36.3**

(c) **T** The pyrogens move from the plasma to affect the hypothalamus and cause fever. The fever recurs at the end of each erythrocytic stage (frequency varies with different species of *Plasmodium*) **36.3**

(d) **T** With virulent infection erythrocyte breakdown can cause excretion of sufficient haem to discolour the urine, hence one local name of 'black water fever' **36.5**

(e) **T** The parasite cannot, however, invade a host without using hepatocytes and erythrocytes; even individuals who are resistant to the cerebral and cardiovascular lesions (the cause of acute death) ultimately suffer chronic damage to spleen and liver with morbidity and shortening of life **36.5**

A382 (a) **F** Primaquines, proguanil and pyrimethamine are active against *Plasmodium* in the exoerythrocytic stages in the liver **36.4, (Fig. 36.1)**

(b) **T** The mechanism of sequestration is unknown but its consequence is that, in the erythrocytic stages, the inhibition of synthesis of plasmodial nucleic acids by quinine is enhanced **36.8– 36.9**

(c) **T** As with quinine and mepacrine, chloroquine is sequestered by infected erythrocytes (see (b)). It binds to plasmodial DNA and inhibits further synthesis of RNA and proteins **36.7**

(d) **F** The order of toxicity of the quinine-like antimalarials is quinine > mepacrine > chloroquine; consequently chloroquine has supplanted quinine except where particular *Plasmodia* have become resistant to the former **36.6, 36.7**

(e) **T** No drug presently available will prevent infection because the sporozoites are resistant to tolerable dosage, but the currently useful antimalarials will control more effectively the contracted disease if the first exoerythrocytic and subsequent erythrocytic stages are impeded by prophylactic use **36.11**

Q383 In amoebic dysentery (intestinal amoebiasis):

(a) infection occurs by ingestion of cysts excreted in the faeces of other hosts
(b) certain antibacterial drugs are of therapeutic use
(c) emetine is an effective therapeutic agent
(d) chloroquine is not as useful as it is in hepatic amoebiasis
(e) metromidazole has proved to be a useful amoebicide

Q384 The anti-protozoal drug(s):

(a) pyrimethamine and sulphadiazine are used concurrently against toxoplasmosis
(b) metronidazole is effective against trichomoniasis (cystitis)
(c) currently available will not cure Chagas' disease (South American trypanosomiasis)
(d) pentamidine is effective against trypanosomiasis
(e) sodium stibogluconate is the drug of choice in the treatment of visceral leishmaniasis

A383 (a) **T** Infections with *Entamoeba histolytica* are prevalent in hot countries with poor sanitation, lack of food hygiene and large populations of flies which carry the cysts on their feet   **36.22**

(b) **T** Ingestion of the cysts results in the establishment of trophozoites in the colon where they feed on gut bacteria; broad-spectrum antibiotics can reduce gut flora to the extent that the trophozoites find inadequate food supplies   **36.25**

(c) **F** Emetine is of little use because inadequate concentrations can be established in the gut at tolerable doses (its cardiotoxicity, amongst other effects, prevents high dosage)   **36.23**

(d) **T** Chloroquine accumulates in the liver and is of use in hepatic amoebiasis (amoebic hepatitis); as with emetine, inadequate intestinal concentrations preclude its use in amoebic dysentery   **36.24**

(e) **T** This drug is active against both hepatic and intestinal amoebiasis and may represent the drug of choice in amoebic dysentery   **36.25**

A384 (a) **T** These drugs kill the endozoites of *Toxoplasma* reducing the spread of infection whilst the immune system of the host reaches full activity against the organism   **36.15**

(b) **T** Orally administered metronidazole is the treatment of choice for trichomoniasis   **36.16**

(c) **T** Chagas' disease is a South American form of trypanosomiasis which is resistant to all known antiprotozoal drugs, though the infection is temporarily suppressed by primaquine and by puromycin   **36.20**

(d) **T** The mechanism of action is unknown, but intramuscular injections of pentamidine are effective against the early (pre-meningoencephalitic) stages of the disease   **36.20**

(e) **T** This form of leishmaniasis (also called kala-azar or black fever) is treated effectively only by sodium stibogluconate or pentamidine, and the former is the more effective   **36.21**

Q385 The anti-helminthic drug:

(a) niridazole is of use in schistosomiasis
(b) bithionol is effective against liver flukes
(c) niclosamide is the drug of choice against several species of tapeworm
(d) diethylcarbamazine is ineffective against filarial worms
(e) thiabendazole has a broad spectrum of activity against roundworm infections

Q386 Cytotoxic drugs used in the therapy of neoplastic diseases include:

(a) cyclophosphamide, which inhibits folic acid synthesis
(b) azathioprine, which acts as a purine antagonist
(c) the alkaloid vinblastine, which interferes with mitotic division
(d) the antibiotic mitomycin, which interferes with pyrimidine synthesis
(e) methotrexate, which inhibits folic acid synthesis

A385 (a) **T** Niridazole has a selective effect on *Schistosoma* flukes 37.17
leading to breakdown of their glycogen stores. The drug
has many side-effects and therapy can be ineffective if
the fluke has produced severe liver damage

(b) **T** The mechanism of action is unknown. The drug is also 37.17
effective against paragonimiasis

(c) **T** It probably acts by inhibiting anaerobic ATP production 37.18
by the worms

(d) **F** Diethylcarbamazine is of use in filariasis, usually in 37.20
conjunction with suramin; the former kills the immature
stages (microfilariae) and the latter the adults

(e) **T** It is inactive against filaria or flatworms. Its mechanism 37.24
of action is unknown

A386 (a) **F** Cyclophosphamide (one of the nitrogen mustards) 38.18
alkylates and cross-links the guanine bases in DNA,
thereby inhibiting replication

(b) **T** Azathioprine is converted to mercaptopurine and sub- 38.18
sequently to the ribose-5-phosphate derivative; the latter
inhibits the formation of 5-phosphoribosylamine (and
thereby interferes with DNA synthesis)

(c) **T** Vinblastine and vincristine interfere with spindle 38.18
formation at metaphase and hence prevent mitotic
division. These drugs also interfere with neurotubule
function and thus can have neurotoxic side-effects

(d) **F** Mitomycin antibiotics form covalent linkages, par- 38.18
ticularly with guanine in DNA. This process of alkylation
prevents DNA replication

(e) **T** Methotrexate (and aminopterin) inhibits the dihydro- 38.18
folate reductase system and thus reduces the production
of tetrahydrofolate. The latter is essential for DNA
synthesis

Q387 The side-effects of cytotoxic drugs may include:

  (a) immunosuppression
  (b) gastrointestinal disturbances
  (c) renal dysfunction
  (d) loss of hair
  (e) inhibition of wound healing

A387 (a) **T** Because cytotoxic drugs have their most marked effects on rapidly dividing cells, the lymphoreticular tissue is markedly affected. Immunosuppression can occur and superinfection may result **38.20**

(b) **T** The gastric and intestinal mucosae have a rapid turnover. Interference with mucosal cell replication may lead to stomatitis, diarrhoea, haemorrhage and septicaemia. Nausea and vomiting are probably due to central nervous effects and are responsive to treatment with anti-emetic phenothiazines **38.20**

(c) **T** Destruction of neoplastic tissue may produce high levels of uric acid in the tubular filtrate. Precipitation of the uric acid in the tubules can cause renal failure **38.20**

(d) **T** Interference with follicular function may lead to cessation of hair growth and shedding of hair. This effect is reversible, and may be offset by application of a tourniquet around the head prior to administration of the drugs **38.20**

(e) **T** Rapid cell division is characteristic of healing tissue; cytotoxic drugs interfere with normal and abnormal cell division **38.20**